8-6-74

PTOMAINE

OTHER BOOKS BY STEWART M. BROOKS:

McBurney's Point: The Story of Appendicitis
The World of the Viruses
The Cancer Story
The V.D. Story
The Sea Inside Us
Civil War Medicine
Our Murdered Presidents: The Medical Story
Basic Biology
Basic Facts of Body Water and Ions
Integrated Basic Science
Basic Science and the Human Body

PTOMAINE

The Story of Food Poisoning

Stewart M. Brooks

SOUTH BRUNSWICK AND NEW YORK: A. S. Barnes and Company
LONDON: Thomas Yoseloff Ltd

A. S. Barnes and Co., Inc.
Cranbury, New Jersey 08512

Thomas Yoseloff Ltd
108 New Bond Street
London W1Y, OQX, England

Library of Congress Cataloging in Publication Data

Brooks, Stewart M
Ptomaine; the story of food poisoning.

Bibliography: p.
1. Ptomaine poisoning. I. Title.
RC143.B76 615.9'54 73-10512
ISBN 0-498-01355-3

PRINTED IN THE UNITED STATES OF AMERICA

to
Dottie and Jay

Contents

Illustrations

* Drawn from an electron micrograph.

A Real-life Preface

One night (at about 10 P.M. to be exact), Joan (a fictitious name to protect the identity of the real victim) was looking for a bedtime snack in the refrigerator when she spotted an unexpected treat behind the carton of milk—three (or was it four?) beautiful, forgotten about, three-day-old shrimp. And Joan ate them. And they were delicious. She went to bed (about 10:45 P.M.) and fell fast asleep. . . . And then all at once (about 2 P.M. or so), all the gastrointestinal devils and demons known to the medical dictionary and mankind came out of nowhere and sank their terrible teeth into Joan's bowels. In a matter of minutes, explosive vomiting, horrendous diarrhea and unbearable pain brought her to the point of collapse and shock and she *hoped* DEATH! But, lo and behold, 36 hours later, Joan was back to normal, saved by no one and nothing but the forces of nature in general and the vagaries of *Staphylococcus aureus* in particular. . . . We shall say much more about *this* and other such upheavals in the pages that follow.

A Real-life Preface

One night [illegible]

[illegible]

Introduction
A Word Is a Word Is a Word

Of the vast list of words that say one thing and mean another—or vice versa—"ptomaine" may very well be at the top. The story goes that an influential Italian toxicologist by the name of Selmi applied the term in 1870 to food poisoning, because in his opinion *ptomaines* were at the root of the problem. And in the context of the times this sounded more than reasonable. After all, ptomaines were the well-recognized end products of protein decay and putrefaction. Moreover, they were exquisitely malodorous. Indeed, this was the reason why these chemical compounds were called ptomaines in the first place—the word coming from the Greek, *ptoma,* meaning carcass or corpse.

And so, for well over fifty years "ptomaine" was the toxicologic gospel of food poisoning, and unto this very day "ptomaine poisoning" (affectionately, "ptomaine") continues to season the language with the scientific naiveté of the past. We now know, to shorten a long story, that ptomaines *do not* cause illness. Smelly food is not necessarily poisonous, and in some cultures putrefied victuals are staples of the diet. Off-tasting food *may* be poisonous, of course, poisonous because of the presence of certain *relatively tasteless* microbes or chemicals or toxins. Tragically, botulinus toxin, the most deadly biological poison known, is *not* unkind to the taste buds. Put otherwise, smelly, off-tasting, *poisonous* food typically represents co-contamination by harmful and harmless substances—the latter serving to warn us of the former. Thus, in a very real sense, Selmi's ptomaines turn out to be our chemical friends.

In both lay and medical circles food poisoning—ptomaine!—denotes, in the classic sense, a sudden, sharp, severe, and short-lived gastrointestinal attack following the intake of food. How long after the intake is typically a matter of hours, but may vary from a few minutes to a couple of days, depending on the *cause,* or etiology, as the doctors say. And the causes are several. In the first place we might overindulge—"too many martinis"; we might be allergic or hypersensitive to certain foods—the "Chinese-restaurant syndrome"; we might unwittingly ingest naturally poisonous "food"—toadstools; we might ingest certain bacteria or their toxins—botulism or salmonellosis; we might ingest a chemical poison as a consequence of an accident—"rat poison instead of baking powder"; and we might conceivably be the victim of an intentional poisoning.

For most intents and purposes, all the many causes of food poisoning fall into one of two major categories—microbial and nonmicrobial. By microbial we mean food poisoning involving microorganisms and/or their toxins. This category, by far and away the more important, accounts for well over 90 percent of all cases of food poisoning. Nonmicrobial poisonings, by contrast, amount to an etiological wastebasket of gastrointestinal disturbances ranging (in incidence) from occasional to rare. As suggested, and for convenience, this book is divided into microbial poisoning (Part One) and nonmicrobial poisoning (Part Two).

PTOMAINE

Part One
MICROBIAL POISONING

1
String Beans

The scene is a cozy little country inn at suppertime. The proprietor, his wife, and three boarders have taken their places at the table and are now passing around the potatoes, bologna, string beans, and the usual bread and butter. The wife is the first to note that the beans are "off," slightly foamy and faintly rancid, a rather irksome finding considering the great care with which she had canned them. In response to her query concerning their edibility one of the boarders suggests a thorough rinsing under cool water. And this is done, but not to the liking of one of the other diners who goes it alone *without* the vegetable. . . . Two days later in this true-life story all four of the "bean eaters" are dead, killed by the most lethal biological poison known to science. An ounce of the stuff could easily extinguish the population of Los Angeles.

We are talking about botulism, the name deriving from the German *Botulismus* and this in turn from the Latin *botulus* (sausage), the etymological point being that most of the early outbreaks occurred in Germany from eating contaminated sausage. The first recorded case dates back to the year 1735. In United States history, the official total number of poisonings is in the neighborhood of 2,000, of which some 1,200 resulted in death. Clearly, the disease is exceptionally rare and exceptionally deadly. In the "great" outbreak of 1963 there were 14 deaths among 46 cases; and to cite a more recent figure, in 1970 5 persons died in an outbreak involving 13 victims. Astonishingly, California leads all other states, accounting for 478 cases out of a total of 1,561 for the span of years from 1899 to 1963.

As already noted in bold relief, botulism is food poisoning in the truest sense of the word, a poisoning caused by a particular toxin* that in turn is produced by a particular bacterial organism called *Clostridium botulinum*—the brother or sister of *Clostridium tetani* (the cause of lockjaw!) and *Clostridium perfringens* (the cause of gas gangrene!)** First isolated by von Emengem in 1895, this organism is a large, rod-shaped bacterial cell (or bacillus) measuring about one micron across and five microns in length. (One micron is equal to 1/25,000 inch.) Clostridia are gram positive (see illustration), motile, and, above all, anaerobic and spore-forming; that is, they pass into a dormant, *heat-resistant* spore stage under adverse environmental conditions—each spore germinating back into the vegetative cell when conditions are just right, especially when there is a lack of oxygen. And a lack of oxygen is encountered in two situations: in the can and in foods (particularly fish) where certain biochemical agents "absorb" oxygen.

Soil is the natural reservoir of clostridial spores, which explains their universal presence and why food processing must either destroy them (via sterilization) at the outset or else provide a chemical environment that prevents their survival and

---

* There are several categories of bacterial toxins, the most dangerous of which are the exotoxins. The botulinus toxin belongs to this group.

** All living things have a two-part scientific name. By convention the "first name" (the genus) is capitalized and the "last name" (the species) is not; both are *italicized.*

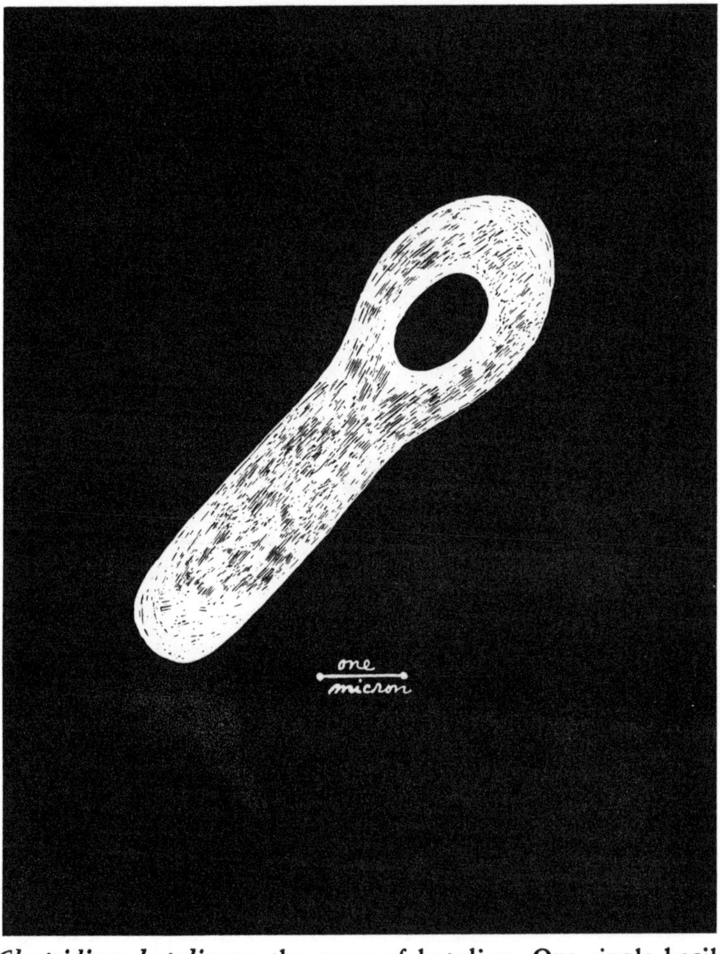

Clostridium botulinum, the cause of botulism. One single bacillus (cell) is shown. Note the spore toward the end and the characteristic way that it causes the cell to bulge. The organism's actual size is indicated by the micron scale.

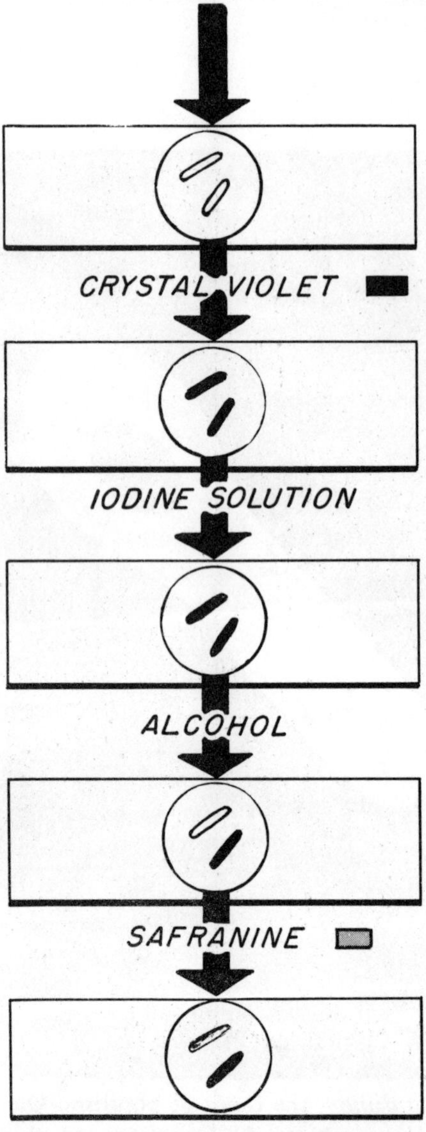

Of great value in the identification of bacteria is gram staining (named in honor of its discoverer Hans Gram). In this illustration two different but look-alike bacterial cells are placed on a glass slide and (1) stained with crystal violet, (2) treated with iodine, (3) *rinsed in alcohol,* (4) counterstained with safranine —*in this order*—and (5) finally examined under the microscope. So-called gram *negative* bacteria (upper cell) are decolorized by alcohol and are thus free to "take" the safranine (red) stain; gram *positive* bacteria are *not* decolorized and thus *retain* the crystal violet stain. As noted in the text, *Clostridium botulinum* is gram positive.

development. Particularly, spores do not survive oxygen, salty solutions, heavy syrups, or high acidity. Were this not so, canned peaches, pickled pigs feet and such would not be with us, at least as we know them. Canned meat and vegetables must always be sterilized at the time of packing. The biggest problem continues to be home-canned food, notably string beans and corn; in more recent years, smoked fish has proved a threat. The cases in the 1963 epidemic ran as follows: 20 involved smoked fish, 2 liver paste, 3 canned tuna fish, 5 home-canned corn, 6 home-canned green beans, 2 home-canned chili peppers, 6 home-canned mushrooms, and 2 home-canned figs.

Clostridium botulinum occurs in six types—A, B, C, D, E, and F—each of which produces its own brand of toxin, the most deadly being A, followed by B. Type A predominates in the soils of the Pacific Coast (hence, the higher mortality in California), while type B predominates in the Mississippi Valley, Great Lakes region, and Atlantic Coast states. These two types and type E are responsible for just about all botulism in this country; type E is associated almost exclusively with smoked or canned fish. Human involvements with types C, D, and F are rare, but not in animals. Forage poisoning in horses and "paralytic disease" in cattle are well recognized problems in Australia and Africa, and here in the U.S. botulism in wild ducks and other waterfowl causes the death of thousands of these birds each year. Further, outbreaks of botulism in chickens (limberneck) are often associated with human cases, these fowl having been fed the toxin-containing food. Experimentally, rabbits, guinea pigs, mice, monkeys, cats, and dogs are susceptible to all six toxin types, whether given orally or by injection.

The six toxins have been studied in great detail. Relative to many bacterial toxins they are *easily* destroyed by heat (boiling for 15 minutes) but highly resistant to the digestive process, even though they are of a protein nature. Indeed, if these toxins were destroyed by digestive juices—like the toxins of diphtheria and tetanus—there would be no botulism! As to their mechanism of poisoning there is now general agreement that they act upon the nerve endings and prevent the release of acetylcholine, the very thing a nerve impulse must do (once it arrives at these endings) in order to contract the muscles. The upshot, of course, is paralysis, and in the language of toxicology these exquisite poisons are dubbed neurotoxins.

With a mortality rate as high as 65 percent, the onset of botulism is one of the most frightening acute encounters known to medicine, in all likelihood topped only by rabies. Typically, the symptoms are abrupt and commence anywhere from 18 to 36 hours after ingestion of the toxin, though the incubation period may vary from four hours to a week or more. Following a very short initial period of lassitude and fatigue, visual disturbances develop, and a loss of acuity and double vision (diplopia) are hallmarks of the poisoning. Too, there is a diminished or total loss of the pupillary reflex; that is, the pupils neither constrict in light nor enlarge in darkness. And the greatest surprise of all, vomiting and diarrhea are *usually* absent; when they are present the cause is probably coincidental contamination rather than the botulinus toxin. The visual disorders now blend in with speech impairment and difficulty in swallowing, which leads to aspiration pneumonia as a result of food or fluid passing into the windpipe. The muscles of the extremities and trunk become weak and eventually a general paralysis ensues; most deaths occur between the second and ninth day, usually from respiratory paralysis or pneumonia. In rare instances, fatalities have occurred during the first day or as late as two weeks or more. And, pathetically, the mind is clear until a short time before death. Among survivors the poisoning usually hits its peak in little over a week and lasts to some degree (namely, visual disturbances) for a couple of months or more. There are, however, no lasting effects.

The diagnosis of botulism relates to the foregoing clinical picture and the simultaneous occurrence of two or more cases following the eating of the same meal. Obviously, the isolated case presents a problem, especially when we consider the several other etiologic possibilities, including myasthenia gravis, encephalitis, poliomyelitis, and atropine poisoning. Laboratory confirmation is made by demonstrating *Clostridium botulinum* or its toxin in the incriminated food or vomitus. Occasionally, the toxin can be demonstrated in the blood. The presence of the toxin in food can be determined by grinding up a sample in a small amount of water, centrifuging the resulting suspension, and then injecting a tiny dose of the supernatant clear fluid into mice—some of the mice being immunized with type A, some with type B, and others with type E *antitoxins.* If *all* the mice die except those given, say, type E antitoxin, this means that the pathogen involved is type E, because *only* type E antitoxin can *neutralize* type E toxin; and the same applies to the other types. This is the only practicable way of distinguishing and identifying the six types of toxin and their respective clostridial producers.

The specific treatment of botulism is far from satisfactory because antitoxins cannot repair the damage *already* done. Nonetheless, because of the possibility that the toxin may still be circulating, antitoxin is given in the hope of preventing further damage. Now available (from the Center for Disease Control, Atlanta, Georgia) is a "trivalent" mixture containing antitoxins A, B, and E. This preparation is preferred over the use of the single antitoxin unless it is definitely known which type toxin is involved. Supportive measures, too, are critically important and may mean the difference between life and death. Water and caloric balance must be maintained, and, in the presence of pharyngeal paralysis (inability to swallow), nutrient fluids are given by vein. Fluid and food by mouth can prove to be dangerous because of the likelihood of aspiration pneumonia. Fur-

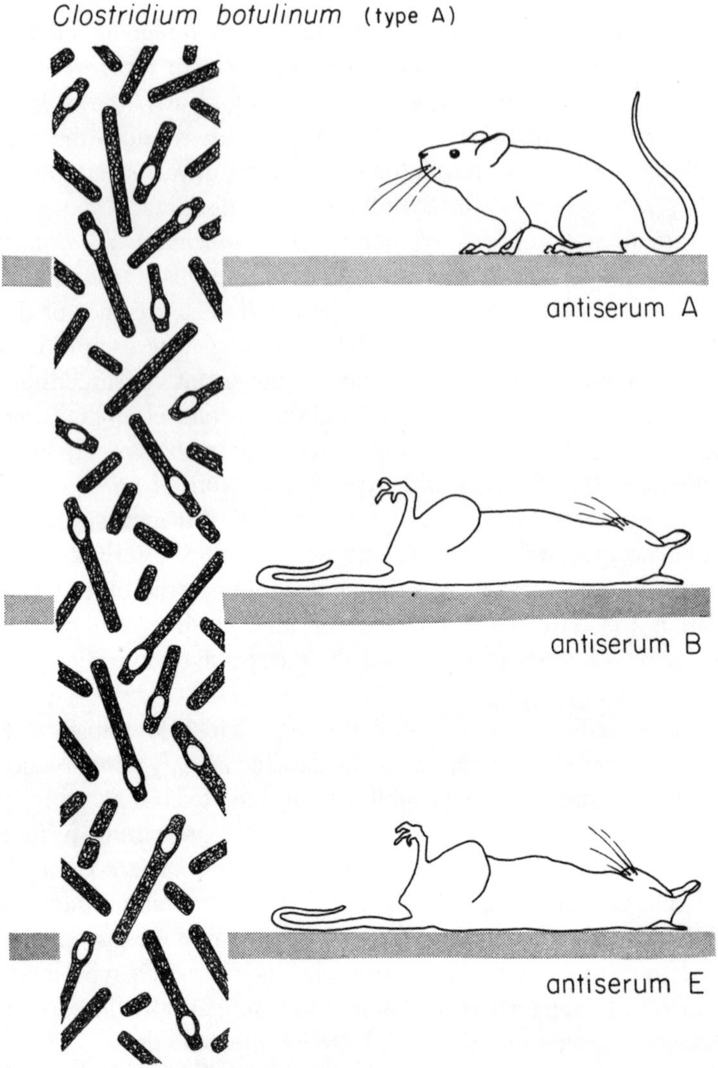

The laboratory procedure shown here is the only way in which we can distinguish among the various types of *Clostridium botulinum.* Type A *antiserum* protects against the toxin of *Clostridium botulinum* type A and type A *only;* and so on.

ther, in the event of severe paralysis, saliva should be aspirated from the throat. The victim should be kept in a darkened room —without visitors—and encouraged to avoid even the slightest unnecessary movement; sedatives may be given to allay anxiety and promote rest. If swallowing becomes impossible a tracheostomy is done, and in the event of cyanosis (bluing of the skin) oxygen is given. Respiratory paralysis calls for the respirator, and in the event of pneumonia the appropriate antibiotic is prescribed.

But if ever an ounce was worth a pound, it is certainly true in the prevention of botulism—in giving antitoxin *before* the onset of signs and symptoms; neutralized while still in the circulation, the toxin is thwarted in its deadly mischief. All exposed persons should be treated *immediately* following appropriate tests for sensitivity to the antitoxin. Almost always such a measure is lifesaving. Also, for the protection of those working with *Clostridium botulinum* in the laboratory, long-lasting active immunity can be achieved by the injection of the toxoids. For example, *formalin-neutralized** type A toxin stimulates the body to produce type A antitoxin, just as tetanus toxoid stimulates the body to produce the appropriate antitoxin against tetanus toxin. Because botulism in man is so rare, however, active immunization is not practiced, which explains the necessity of administering a big dose of "ready-made" antitoxin to exposed persons (*passive* immunity). (The use of toxoids here would be of no avail for the very simple reason that it takes *time* for the body to respond.) Interestingly, active immunization has been carried out in lower animals when economically feasible. In Australia, botulism of sheep and cattle has assumed sufficient proportions to justify small-scale efforts in this direction.

* Formalin (formaldehyde) chemically neutralizes toxins to produce so-called *harmless* toxoids.

The real answer to botulism in man, though, lies in the destruction of the organism and its spores in the processing of food or, at the very least, in creating a chemical environment in which they cannot survive. And from a public health point of view, food processing in general and canning in particular must zero in on *Clostridium botulinum.* An improperly processed can of corn, for example, could very well turn out to be a lethal can—and it is indeed lethal if clostridial spores are present. If thousands of such cans of corn are involved the outcome could be catastrophic.

Through the efforts of the National Canners Association and United States Public Health Service, commercial canning has become an exact science and botulism at this level has just about been reduced to zero. For every type of canned food and for every step along the way, the laboratory and production are in constant touch to insure the annihilation of *Clostridium botulinum* and its spores. Special attention, of course, is directed to nonsalty, neutral foods—namely, meats and vegetables—in which the spores are most likely to germinate and produce toxin. Here, sufficient heat must be employed to destroy every single spore that happens to be present. Such temperatures are precisely known, and to be on the safe side—exceeded! Frozen foods, too, have an excellent safety record but the consumer must be on his guard. In point of fact, frozen foods that have been allowed to thaw and stored at 50°F. or above may give rise to botulinus toxin in the event spores are present. Once thawed, frozen foods must be used right away!

Today, home-canned products are responsible for the bulk of botulism, and those who engage in this gastronomic art are understandably playing with fire unless they know about *Clostridium botulinum*—and its spores—and its deadly toxin! Especially dangerous are nonsalty, nonsyrupy, nonacid preparations —notably meats and vegetables. Unless the spores are destroyed

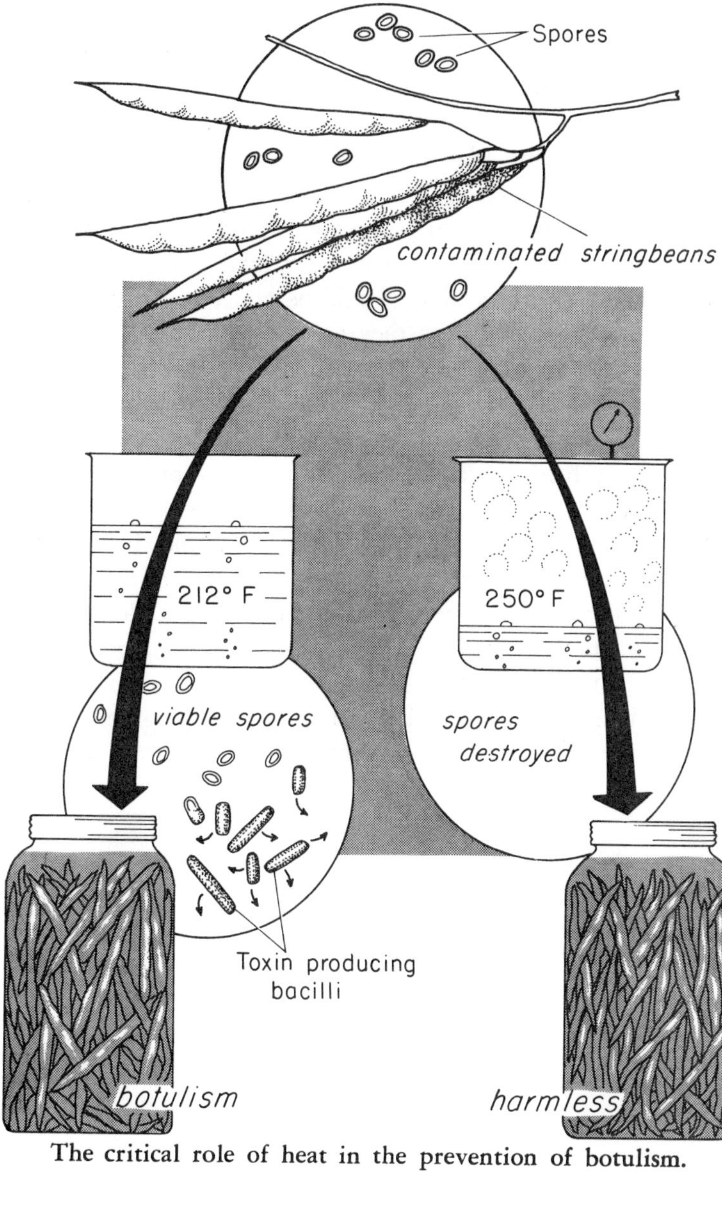

The critical role of heat in the prevention of botulism.

in such foods they will germinate in the *air-free* conditions of the jar and more than likely kill somebody. Spores are resistant, as we know, and may survive long periods of boiling (212°F.). The pressure cooker (250°F.) is the only answer for meat, vegetables, and the like, but even here the housewife must follow directions carefully and pay special attention to the temperature and timing; equally important, the food must be fresh and thoroughly washed and clean. As a final precaution, home-canned meats and vegetables should be boiled (and thoroughly stirred) ten minutes before they are served or even tasted by the cook, the ten minutes commencing at the onset of boiling, not before. If the toxin is present, this will destroy it.

Finally, damaged canned food should never be used and most certainly any food displaying the least evidence of spoilage discarded. Although botulinus toxin and spoilage are not necessarily associated with each other, many authorities believe that toxin-containing foods are never *entirely* normal in appearance, odor, or taste. Unfortunately, there are degrees of tolerance and sensitivity among different persons, and "damaged goods" are indeed eaten, often with gusto in the instance of exotic foods. Be that as it may, if something tastes "off," the slightest bit off —especially the vegetables—for heaven's sake, SPEAK UP!

2
Cream Puffs

From the Greek word for berry, *kokkos,* comes "coccus," which may be defined conveniently as a *spherical* bacterial cell. For the most part, cocci measure slightly less than one micron across, or about one-tenth the diameter of a red blood cell. Like all bacteria they reproduce asexually by splitting in two (fission), and the typical configurations assumed by the daughter cells serve to relegate them into rather distinct categories—notably, diplococci, streptococci ("strep") and staphylococci ("staph"). Diplococci, as the prefix suggests, occur in pairs; strep occur in twisted chains (from the Greek *streptos,* twisted); and staph occur in grapelike clusters (from the Greek *staphule,* bunch of grapes). All staph are gram positive.

The great majority of cocci (like people) are good guys, but the bad guys are really bad. To illustrate the latter, *Diplococcus pneumoniae* is a common cause of pneumonia; *Streptococcus pyogenes* causes rheumatic fever; and the pathogen *Staphylococcus aureus* causes all kinds of trouble such as pimples, boils, abscesses, carbuncles, tonsillitis, osteomyelitis, and similar pus-forming lesions. Indeed, pus is the hallmark of staph infections and none other than the material in which these organisms were first observed by Louis Pasteur in the year 1880. And central to our concern here is the fact that *Staphylococcus aureus* is probably the most common cause of food poisoning. Since "staphylococcal food poisoning," to use the official designation, is not reportable, however, the number of cases occurring annually is unknown. One educated guess puts the figure at well over five million cases per year. The ailment strikes most persons at one time or another during their lives, though no great attention is paid to it unless large groups of people are attacked. The bakery, church supper, and college mess hit the front page, but seldom if ever does the midnight snack merit publicity.

Staph food poisoning is an interplay of three basic factors—the right strain of *Staphylococcus aureus,* the right kind of food, and the right temperature. For all intents and purposes, this equation dates back only to 1930, but the poisoning proper—or what we have excellent reason to take as staph poisoning—must be at least as old as recorded history. Actually, a chronologic sampling of the medical literature on the subject affords a fascinating view of a very hazy picture eventually coming into focus.

The first breakthrough pointing to the true cause of the poisoning came in 1884, four years following Pasteur's discovery of the microbe in pus. Three hundred cases of cheese poisoning in Michigan that year prompted the public health people to call in a Professor Victor Vaughan and a Doctor George Sternberg. Working independently, Vaughan in Michigan and Sternberg at Johns Hopkins University, these investigators demonstrated the presence of staphylococci and a potent poison. Interestingly—and significantly—animals were found to be *resistant* to both. Professor Vaughan purposely poisoned himself with alcohol extracts of the cheese and a Doctor Duggan, who assisted Sternberg, actually ate a half ounce of the incriminated food. Three hours later he (Duggan) was attacked

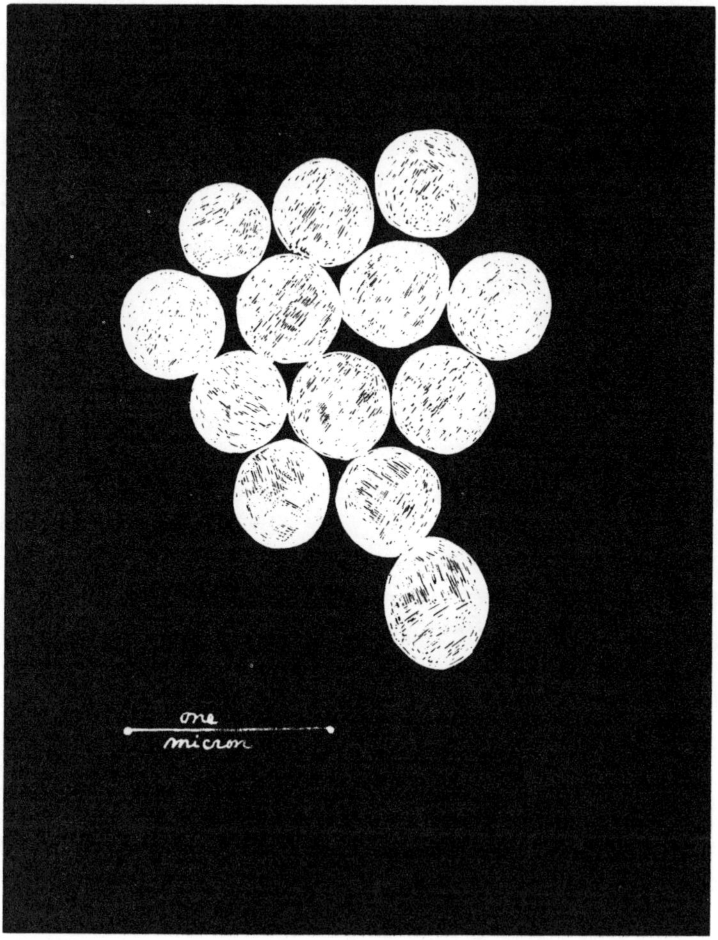

Staphylococcus aureus, the cause of staphylococcal food poisoning. Note the grapelike cluster of spherical cells (cocci).

by nausea, vomiting, and diarrhea. Professor Vaughan in *Public Health Papers and Reports* (1884) concluded, "that the poisonous material, whatever it may be, is contained in the alcohol extract. This would indicate a chemical poison and not a bacteric one. However, this chemical poison might be *generated by the agency of bacteria.*" (Italics mine.) And more to the point still, Sternberg remarks: "It seems not improbable that the *poisonous principle* (italics mine) is a ptomaine developed in the cheese as a result of the vital activity of micrococci [staphylococci]."

Although these revelations were repeatedly confirmed here and abroad (one report actually tracing an epidemic to a particular cow with staph mastitis), staph food poisoning was not officially christened until 1930 (in the *Journal of Preventive Medicine*), at which time G. M. Dack and his co-workers cultured a "yellow hemolytic staphylococcus" from a poisonous—but delicious!—three-layer Christmas cake, complete with thick cream filling, icing, maraschino cherries, and pistachio nuts. A little less than an ounce of "toxic filtrate" (cell-free culture medium in which the staph was grown) produced severe poisoning in one human volunteer, and less than a half ounce produced mild poisoning in two others.

Staphylococcus aureus is easily cultured in the laboratory; blood-containing media produce luxuriant growths of golden colonies, hence the designation "aureus." But as indicated earlier not all strains of *Staphylococcus aureus* cause food poisoning. In almost all cases, apparently, the troublemakers are hemolytic (destroying red blood cells) and coagulase positive (clot blood plasma)—effects produced by the release of the toxin hemolysin and enzyme coagulase, respectively. Interestingly, though, these two agents play little or no role in staph poisoning, the real cause of which is another toxin dubbed "enterotoxin."* Unfor-

* The term enterotoxin is often applied to *any* bacterial toxin specific for the intestinal lining. *Staph* enterotoxin is the best known and the most potent.

tunately, there is presently no sure way of detecting enterotoxin except in the human volunteer, for most animals are singularly resistant. Monkeys and kittens can be made ill, but the dose is way above what it takes to put a human out of commission. In sum, then, poison staph release an enterotoxin and *almost* always hemolysin and coagulase; the latter can be demonstrated easily in the laboratory. *Absolute* proof of identity obviously calls for the human volunteer.

Staph enterotoxin is soluble and unlike most other potent bacterial toxins relatively resistant (thermostable) to high temperatures. Nonetheless, heating may effect considerable detoxication. In one experiment, the same amount of enterotoxin boiled for 30 minutes and 60 minutes poisoned 4 out of 15 and 2 out of 14 monkeys, respectively. When subjected to steam under pressure (autoclaved) at 250°F. for 20 minutes the same dose poisoned only one out of 14 monkeys.

The conditions necessary for an outbreak of staph poisoning are, as already indicated, well recognized—to wit, an enterotoxin-producing staph, a suitable food, and the right temperature (improper storage). Stated otherwise, when the right staph encounters the right food at the right temperature for the right length of time, sufficient reproduction (growth) ensues to yield poisonous levels of enterotoxin. This, of course, begs the question: How much enterotoxin does it take to cause trouble? Or, put a little differently: Do individuals vary in their susceptibility to enterotoxin? And the answer is yes, definitely. For example, in one experiment, eight drops of filtrate of an enterotoxic staph culture caused poisoning in one human volunteer, whereas a half ounce caused no signs or symptoms at all in another volunteer. And at the clinical level, of 325 people who ate an incriminated food, "only" 195 were sick and, as we would expect, some more than others. Quite logically, therefore, the *severity* of staph food poisoning depends on the size

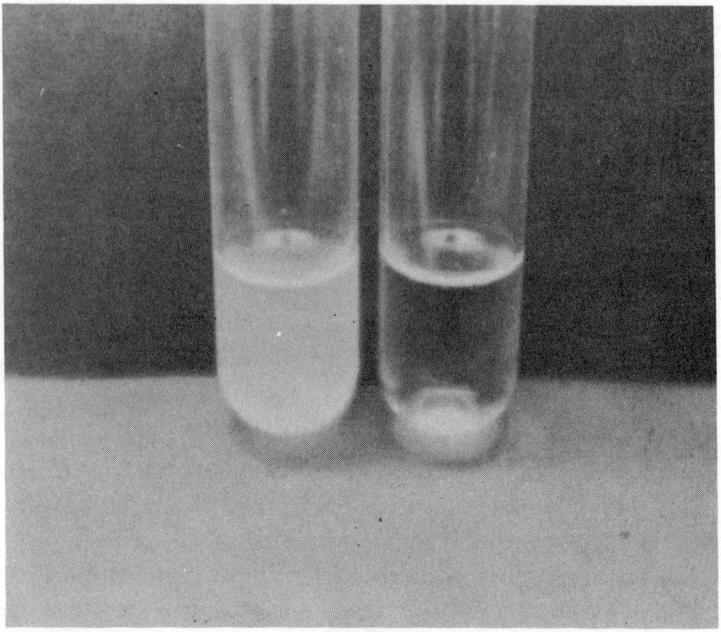

The staph responsible for food poisoning secrete hemolysin, a toxin that causes the destruction of red cells (hemolysis). In the experiment shown here, hemolytic staph were added to a few drops of blood suspended in water (right). Compare with the *cloudy control* tube to the left. Though hemolysin plays no role in the actual poisoning, it aids in identification and diagnosis.

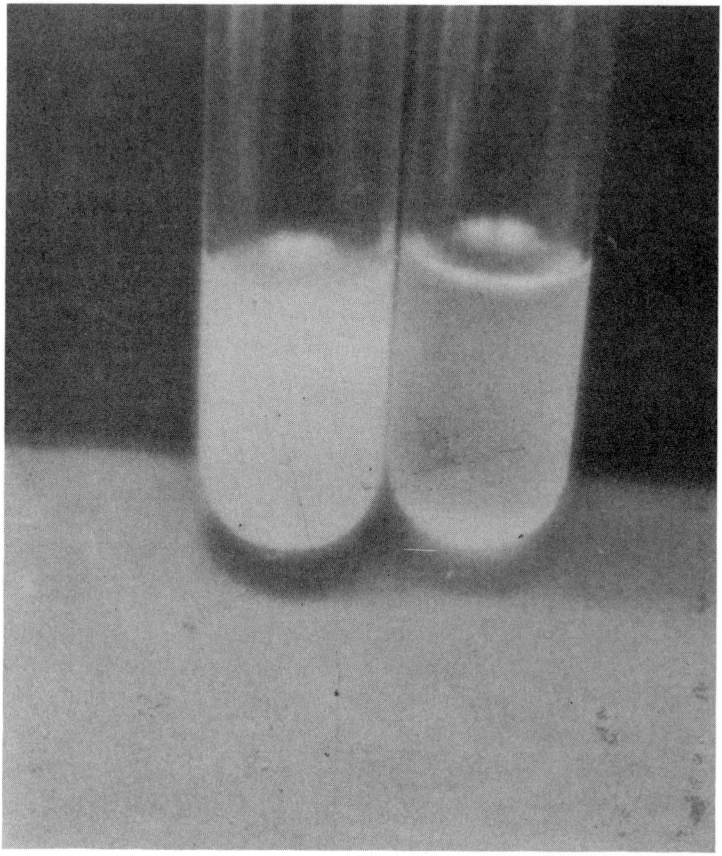

The *particular* staph causing food poisoning secretes coagulase, an enzyme that causes the *clotting* of blood serum (tube to the left—coagulase positive). Tube to the right shows *no* clotting (coagulase negative). Though coagulase, like hemolysin, plays no role in the actual poisoning, it aids in identification and diagnosis.

of the dose of enterotoxin and on the degree of susceptibility.

Staphylococci, to say about the least, are ubiquitous and may be cultured (isolated) from almost any source—air, soil, water, food, milk, and, most especially, the human body. And, comparatively speaking, they are hardy, much more so than other cocci; many strains show surprising resistance to heat, germicides, and other physical and chemical agents. The nose and mouth and skin are usually teeming with staph, which means that the butcher, the baker, the cook, the waiter, the housewife —*food handlers*—contaminate what we eat. They really contaminate what we eat in the event the staph are enterotoxin producers, and according to some authorities about half of normal individuals harbor such microbial malefactors. These people are obviously the most insidious purveyors of staph poisoning because they are seldom identified, and when they are the Pepto-Bismol is well beyond its last drop. In one classic outbreak involving poisoned cream puffs, the responsible germ was traced to the nose and throat of the healthy baker who harbored the strain for a good year in spite of medical treatment. Persons with pyogenic (pus-forming) infections—abscesses, boils, carbuncles, and the like—almost always harbor *Staphylococcus aureus,* and almost always the various strains involved are enterotoxic. But at least in these cases there is a warning! In short, nearly all cases of staph poisoning can be traced to human carriers who come into contact with food. Occasionally, an outbreak can be traced to milk and dairy products contaminated with staph of bovine origin.

The next logical condition to be considered in our toxic equation is the food itself. It is one thing for a staphylococcus to encounter food that it does not like and quite another to encounter food that it does like—a situation, other things being equal, leading to a population explosion and the production of poisonous quantities of enterotoxin. Put another way, even the most virulent strains do not cause trouble unless they multiply. Equally important and significant, a population explosion can ensue *without* signs of spoilage, and in the majority of cases the poisoned food is palatable. . . . How fortunate it would be if enterotoxin insulted the taste bud the way it insults the intestine.

Cream and custard-filled bakery goods—rich pastries—are responsible for the greatest number of poisonings, probably followed by ham and cheddar cheese. Other foods and dishes pinpointed in poisonings and outbreaks include custards, milk, processed meats, fish, poultry, tongue, dried beef, sausage, sandwich spreads, potato salad, chicken salad, chicken gravy, chicken à la king, creamed chicken, creamed salmon, creamed tuna, ice cream, bread pudding, and hollandaise sauce.

And now for the temperature. Over 42°F., as a rule of thumb, staph multiply in food, the extent of the growth depending on the elevation above this figure, the time over which the temperature operates (incubation period) and, of course, the nature of the food. In one typical laboratory experiment, chicken à la king and ham salad were *inoculated* with staph and incubated at 50°F. for 24 hours. Whereas the ham salad *remained* at a staphylococcal count of one million (cells per gram of salad), the chicken à la king rose from one to 50 million during this period. At 95°F. the counts for similarly inoculated samples of the ham salad and chicken à la king rose (in 24 hours) to 10 million and 100 million, respectively. Clearly, in this experiment anyway, chicken à la king proved more dangerous than ham salad at 95°F., and *much* more dangerous than ham at 50°F. Further, ham salad or chicken à la king or any other staph-prone food becomes more and more poisonous the longer it stands around unrefrigerated or improperly refrigerated. In a typical case at an army camp, sliced ham served at the noon mess felled 50 soldiers within four hours after eating; the same ham served the following morning felled 300 in one hour!

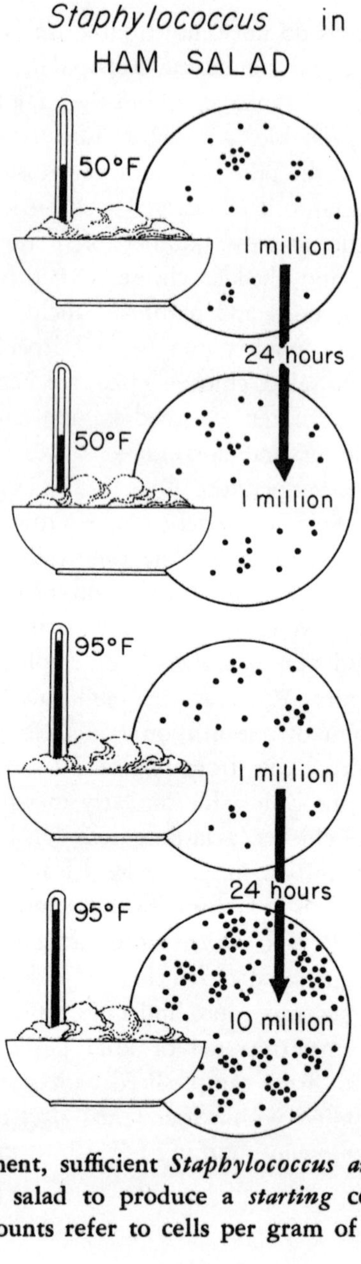

In this experiment, sufficient *Staphylococcus aureus* was inoculated into ham salad to produce a *starting* cell count of *one* million. (All counts refer to cells per gram of salad.)

Staphylococcus in
CHICKEN A LA KING

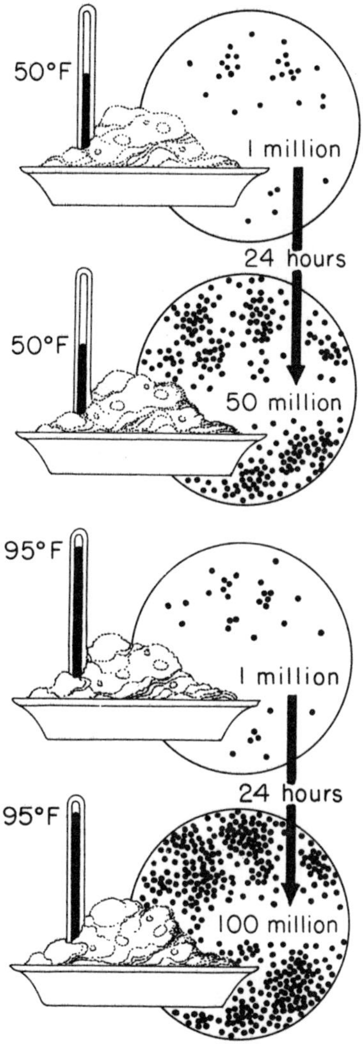

In this experiment sufficient *Staphylococcus aureus* was inoculated into chicken à la king to produce a starting cell count of one million. (All counts refer to cells per gram of food.)

Staph food poisoning is almost never fatal, although its victims have been said to wish that it were. In the typical case salivation, the first sign, usually appears in 2 to 4 hours, followed by nausea, vomiting, diarrhea, retching, abdominal cramps, sweating, headache, and prostration. There is no fever. Symptoms persist for 3 to 6 hours and recovery is usually complete in a day or two. In mild cases nausea and vomiting may occur without diarrhea, or there may be cramps and diarrhea without vomiting. In really severe cases blood may appear in stools and vomitus, the blood pressure may drop precipitously, and shock may even occur; some victims require hospitalization and may not be out of the woods for a week or so. A few fatal cases have occurred in the young, aged, and debilitated. In one well-publicized episode, two children died within 24 hours after drinking a glass of goat's milk from an animal with staph mastitis.

The diagnosis of staph poisoning is basically an accessory after the fact, but nevertheless a vital link in public health affairs; that is, the victims are up and about again a day or two before the cream-cocoanut pie yields a culture of *Staphylococcus aureus.* Actually, though, the clinical situation usually affords a speedy presumptive diagnosis. Sudden onset *plus* brief symptoms *plus* rapid recovery equals staphylococcal food poisoning. Further, the patient is usually one of a number of similarly affected individuals. The laboratory report, in other words, is typically confirmatory.

Commonly, detective work is involved in tracing down the postulated pathogen. If a list of foods served at the previous meal is available, various items can be tabulated for those made ill as well as for those who were not ill, and in this fashion a common denominator arrived at—for example, a food with an unrefrigerated history. And from this food the laboratory people must not only isolate *Staphylococcus aureus,* but also demonstrate the strain to be hemolytic, coagulase positive, and if possible, poisonous to monkeys or man. The human volunteer, we shall recall, affords the only absolute means of putting the finger on staph enterotoxin. Finally, it is now possible via "phage typing" to pinpoint the *precise strain* of enterotoxic staph involved and thereby the source. For example, if strain "so and so" isolated from our cream-cocoanut pie turns out to match the strain isolated from the nose of the baker, then science has indeed performed an ultimate in epidemiology.

In way of treatment there is no specific drug or serum of value. *The Merck Manual of Diagnosis and Therapy* stresses bed rest and, hardly as a surprise, "convenient access to bathroom, commode, or bedpan." Further, intravenous infusions of glucose and saline solutions are given to manage dehydration in the face of protracted vomiting and blood or "plasma expander" is given in severe cases when shock is impending. Vomiting can usually be controlled by sedation with phenobarbital or by injections of antiemetics, such as Dramamine or Compazine; diarrhea usually yields to paregoric, Lomotil, or Donnagel. The latter is a popular prescription item of some merit. Its belladonna alkaloids slow down the intestine; its phenobarbital, as indicated, quietens the vomiting center, and its kaolin and pectin purportedly adsorb and detoxify staphylococcal enterotoxin. Nothing is permitted by mouth so long as nausea and vomiting persist, and when they do cease, tea, cereal, or bouillon with added salt may be taken. Once warm liquids are tolerated, the diet may be increased gradually to include such bland foods as cooked gelatin, jellied consommé, simple puddings, and soft-boiled eggs.

Staph poisoning, by way of repetition, centers on the multiplication of enterotoxic staphylococci within food during the interval between preparation and consumption, and its prevention clearly centers on preventing this multiplication. Putting first things first, staph should be avoided and excluded from food, and this means strict personal cleanliness on the part of cooks and bakers. It certainly means weeding out food handlers with abscesses, boils, carbuncles, pus-forming lesions, and other staph infections. But staphylococci are everywhere, as we know, and even the most rigorous standards cannot assure the safety of unrefrigerated perishable foods. A top-notch bakery can turn out a top-notch—and harmless—cream puff only to have it encounter staph; and this could well mean trouble unless A) it is eaten right away or B) it is properly refrigerated. If it does encounter enterotoxic staph and if it is left around at room temperatures, multiplication ensues and enough enterotoxin is generated to produce poisoning. Laboratory studies have demonstrated that such a cream puff (and other staph-prone foods) may become dangerous in eight to ten hours, but typically there is no off-flavor or taste. Contrariwise, even though other conditions necessary for poisoning are fulfilled, enterotoxin *is not* formed in periods up to four weeks where food is kept at the *proper temperatures.*

Low temperatures (−100°F. and below) do not destroy staphylococci and in one study 50 strains were isolated from frozen vegetables, a dozen of which were enterotoxic. For this very reason thawed-out frozen foods must be used right away, and the package tells us so. Actually, the warning should be in much larger type than it is. Refreezing certainly stops staphylococcal multiplication, but it certainly does not detoxify any enterotoxin that may have been generated during the thaw. By and large, frozen foods (including ice cream!) are staph problems only if the consumer makes them so, and the same applies to just about all commercial food products. The ready-cured ham, to cite a classic example, is typically enterotoxin-free when purchased but readily becomes poisonous when permitted to smolder away at room temperatures.

To summarize, our hands are more or less tied when it comes to eradicating staph; that is, like mosquitos, they are part of the environment. But, what we can do is to prevent them from *multiplying* and producing enterotoxin in food during the interval between purchase or preparation and consumption. Except at mealtime, perishables belong in the refrigerator! And to be on the safe side A) periodically check the refrigerator temperature and B) do not stretch your luck even at 41°F., particularly with staph-prone foods and dishes (p. 39). The week-old chicken gravy is *probably* all right, but then again. . . . And do not forget the freezer—it should be freezing!

3
Chicken

The very same year (1880) Louis Pasteur in France discovered the staphylococcus, Karl Eberth in Germany found the typhoid bacillus in the lymph glands and spleen of persons dying from typhoid fever. Bacillus in Latin means "little rod," and this is exactly what the cause of typhoid fever looks like under the microscope—rod-shaped bacterial cells arranged every which way and, in the living condition, swimming actively about via long, hairlike appendages. And in contrast to both staph and clostridia, typhoid bacilli are gram negative. But as history and nature would have it the typhoid bacillus turned out to be *structurally indistinguishable* from countless other bacilli; indeed, the typhoid bacillus turned out to be a member of an enormously large tribe of bacteria now labeled "salmonellae" (in honor of Daniel Salmon, the American pathologist who first described a member of the group in 1885). Presently about 600 species are recognized, all with the official first name (genus) of *Salmonella.* For example, the typhoid bacillus bears the scientific name, *Salmonella typhi.*

Salmonellae inhabit the intestinal tract of man and animals and an estimated 0.2 percent of the population are asymptomatic carriers, that is, individuals who harbor the organisms *without* manifestation of infection. Some are carriers for life, particularly food handlers working with uncooked meat and carcasses. Virtually all domestic and wild animals have been shown to harbor salmonellae, with infection rates ranging from 1 to 50 percent. And the kernel of salmonella infection, or salmonellosis, as the doctors say, is that the organisms are passed in the feces and almost always enter a new host via ingestion, usually as contaminated milk, food, or water. To put it bluntly, salmonellosis is essentially a fecal-oral situation.

The nature of the infection—if indeed infection ensues—depends on the species in question. Speaking generally, there are two kinds of salmonellosis—one a typhoidal involvement in which the causative organism makes its way into the blood in the *initial* stage of the disease (and the symptoms are systemic and widespread) and the other an acute gastroenteritis in which only a very small number of patients display bacteremia (bacteria in the blood). More particularly, *Salmonella typhi* and *Salmonella paratyphi* cause, respectively, typhoid and paratyphoid fever (similar to typhoid but not as serious), and countless other species cause acute gastroenteritis—or food poisoning. Also, whereas *Salmonella typhi* and *Salmonella paratyphi* are peculiar to man, the food-poisoning species relate to both man and animals. In other words, man and animals, especially animals, are the *reservoirs* of infection and must be taken into account in any program that concerns itself with the control of salmonellosis. And here it is important to point out that although typhoid and paratyphoid fever upon *occasion* are associated with contaminated food and acute gastroenteritis, they are seldom considered in the framework of salmonella food poisoning. Further, and for our purpose, salmonellosis and salmonella food poisoning are synonymous.

And it is equally important to take note of the inaccuracy of the expression "poisoning," notwithstanding its solid entrenchment in medical as well as lay circles. In point of fact, salmonellosis is an *infection* of the gastrointestinal tract, whereas staph food poisoning and botulism are indeed true poisonings (or intoxications) resulting from the ingestion of *toxins* present in food. Thus, *bacteriologically* speaking, food poisoning is a matter of food intoxication *or* food infection; almost all cases of the former relate to staph and almost all cases of the latter relate to salmonella organisms. Coming right down to the basic pathology of the situation, then, the acute gastroenteritis of staphylococcal food poisoning stems from the action of enterotoxin (on the intestinal lining) and the acute gastroenteritis of salmonellosis stems from the multiplication of bacterial cells (*infection!*).

This brings to the fore a major clinical distinction among food poisonings with respect to what is called the incubation period, or the time between the entrance of an infecting organism into the body and the *first* appearance of the symptoms consequent to its multiplication. Strictly speaking, staph poisoning and botulism have no incubation period because they are not infections. Still, the expression is applied to these intoxications and in this context means the only thing it can mean—the time it takes the toxins to cause trouble. For staph, as we know, this is about three hours. Salmonellosis, on the other hand, has an average incubation period—a *true* incubation period—of some 12 hours, with a range of 6 to 48 hours.

To backtrack historically for a moment, the first reported outbreak of salmonellosis occurred in 1888 in Frankenhausen, Germany. A total of 57 persons were stricken from eating contaminated beef and one died two days later. The famous bacteriologist August Gärtner isolated a microbe from the organs of this victim and also the same organism from the diseased cow. He christened the pathogen *Bacillus enteritidis* and others were soon to dub it Gärtner's bacillus. A few years later another outbreak occurred in Belgium, this time from contaminated sausage, and once again *Bacillus enteritidis* was isolated from the victims. Moreover, the organism was shown to be "poisonous" to mice, rats, guinea pigs, rabbits, and dogs. Eventually, *Bacillus enteritidis* was found to belong to the salmonellae and officially named *Salmonella enteritidis*. Today, though, the prevailing pathogen of salmonellosis, in the United States anyway, is *Salmonella typhimurium*. Runner-up species (in the United States) are *S. newport* (to abbreviate), *S. montevideo, S. oranienburg, S. choleraesuis, S. schottmueller,* and *S. anatum,* in order of decreasing frequency.

Any item of food or drink may be contaminated directly or indirectly with salmonellae from human or animal carriers. Although the human carrier is certainly of epidemiologic importance, present evidence points to the enormous animal reservoir as the major source of disease, particularly poultry and eggs. Pork, beef, and lamb probably rank next, with raw meats purchased in retail markets showing contamination rates ranging from 1 to 60 percent, depending on the geographical area. Other recognized "source items" are the numerous by-products of the meat packaging industry—bone meal, fertilizer, animal foods, and the like. Contaminated poultry and meats not only cause infection but also serve to spread salmonellae to previously uncontaminated products via utensils, tables, and other items in the processing plant, market, or kitchen. Not uncommonly, a salmonella outbreak can be traced to an otherwise clean meat slicer. And as for eggs the situation is a "sitting duck." Salmonellae may contaminate the external shell—hence, the problem of cracked eggs—or actually appear in the yolk in the event the hen suffers ovarian salmonellosis. Understandably, the matter is substantially made worse in the pooling of large numbers for freezing or drying; that is, the one bad egg may easily poison the whole batch.

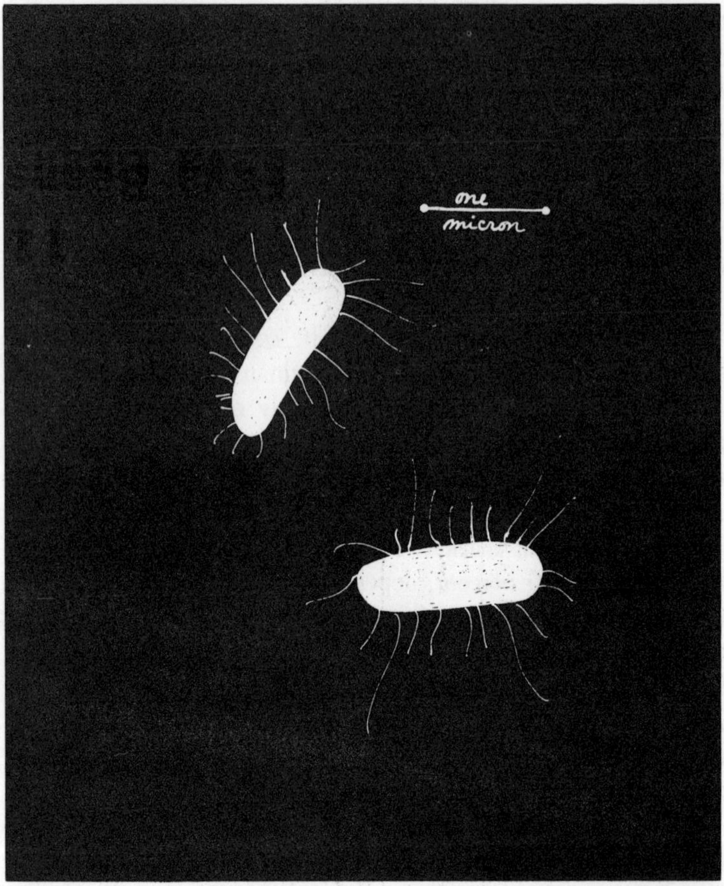

Salmonella typhimurium, a common cause of salmonellosis. Two bacterial cells (bacilli) are shown. Note the flagella responsible for the organism's motility.

The common occurrence of salmonellae in food makes contact with these organisms almost inevitable. In the United States, there are approximately two million cases of salmonellosis annually, excluding the thousands of Americans not seen by a physician. The infections kill about 60 each year. Dr. Henry Bauer of the Minnesota State Department of Health cites six major factors involved in today's salmonella problem: We are eating in restaurants more frequently than ever before and, even at home, are more likely to consume mass-produced foods (meaning the average diet contains ingredients from a variety of subsidiary suppliers, each additional supplier being another potential source of salmonellae); pet food tends to be mass produced, and sometimes "fortified" with highly salmonella-contaminated material from rendering plants; rapid, inexpensive transportation means that foods—including contaminated foods—can be conveyed great distances; food-processing equipment is not always properly designed for sanitary maintenance; there is no satisfactory antibody test for telling which one of the 1,300 or so salmonella seratypes is involved in a given outbreak; and finally, no vaccines are available (except for typhoid and paratyphoid fever). Also, there is a certain indifference at both the public and professional levels, relatively speaking anyway. Salmonellosis is not a fashionable disease like the flu, or, as Dr. Bauer puts it, "Who sits around the dinner table and talks about his bowel movements?"

As a rule of thumb, contact with a pathogenic microorganism does not in itself insure the establishment of infection. In the first place, the invader may not be in sufficient number, and in the second place the host may be resistant. And in the instance of salmonellosis there is the additional factor of species multiplicity, some, as noted previously, causing typhoidal infections, some acute gastroenteritis, and others inapparent, or asymptomatic, infection. For example, *Salmonella anatum* usually produces acute gastroenteritis and only rarely invades the bloodstream, while *Salmonella choleraesuis* usually invades the bloodstream and only rarely produces acute gastroenteritis. The number of salmonella organisms it takes to produce infection is not known, although it is thought to be large, probably in the vicinity of 100,000 (based on a few experiments involving human volunteers).

And often overlooked is host resistance, a factor which may well spell the difference between infection and noninfection (or at least inapparent infection). Or to put it another way, the right species in the right number may poison some and not others. The right species in the right number is especially likely to attack individuals who are missing a part of the stomach (as a result of subtotal gastrectomy) because they lack hydrochloric acid, a bactericidal agent par excellence. Again, animal studies have shown that antibiotics may upset the immunologic applecart by killing off the normal microbes of the intestine, which normally compete with and suppress ingested troublemakers. In one experiment, antibiotics increased the susceptibility of mice to infection with *Salmonella typhi* 100,000 fold! Additionally, a number of diseases are known to predispose to salmonellosis, including certain tumors, cirrhosis, leukemia, sickle-cell anemia, and a strange infection called bartonellosis (prevalent in Peru and Bolivia). According to one source, four out of ten patients with bartonellosis may come down with salmonellosis.

The pathologic mechanism at the root of salmonellosis is the multiplication of salmonellae among the cells composing the mucosa (lining) of the gastrointestinal tract. Dead salmonellae do not produce food poisoning, and this has been demonstrated over and over again in human volunteers. Consequent to this multiplication the mucosa becomes red and swollen and tiny hemorrhages often occur; the upshot is a fulminating gastroenteritis. The incubation period varies from 6 to 48 hours, with an average time, as mentioned earlier, of 12 hours, considerably longer than the "incubation period" in staph poisoning. The onset, nonetheless, is abrupt with nausea, vomiting, abdominal cramps, severe diarrhea, and prostration accompanied by headache, chills, and fever. In severe cases blood may appear in the vomitus and stools and the victim may go into shock as a result of dehydration (that is, the loss of fluid lowers the blood volume and thereby the blood pressure). The loss of fluid further entails a loss of acid from the stomach and alkali (base) from the intestine, and this may plunge the body into an acid-base imbalance, the "direction" of the imbalance depending on the predominating loss. If more acid than alkali is lost the upshot is alkalosis; if more alkali than acid is lost the upshot is acidosis. Other vital elements lost in the vomitus and stools include "electrolytes" (namely, sodium and potassium). Usually the illness lasts from 24 to 48 hours, but an occasional victim will have symptoms for as long as two weeks or more. The case-fatality rate rarely exceeds 1 percent, with almost all deaths occurring in infants, the aged, and in persons with major underlying disease. About half the patients continue to pass the causative organism during the second week after the onset and about 10 percent display positive stools at the end of six months. The very few still positive at the end of one year are labeled chronic carriers.

The diagnosis of salmonellosis on a clinical basis is difficult in the individual case because of the many other possible kinds of acute gastroenteritis, including staph food poisoning. When the victim is one of a group that becomes ill after eating a certain food, however, and when the symptoms are typical, the diagnosis is generally easy. Once again, as with staph and botulism, the food may disclose no evidence of contamination. Diagnosis is aided by the finding of the bacteria in food, vomitus, feces, blood, or urine, and also by the appearance in the blood of agglutinins; the latter are antibodies that cause the clumping together, or agglutination, of the causative organism. For example, if the patient's blood agglutinates a suspension of *Salmonella typhimurium,* this particular species is thereby pinpointed as the cause. Further, highly refined agglutination tests are available in state and federal laboratories to go beyond the species level and pinpoint strains, for example, to pinpoint a particular strain of *Salmonella typhimurium.* Actually, the identification of species and strains is a sine qua non in the public health surveillance of salmonellosis.

The treatment of salmonellosis is essentially the same as in staph food poisoning, the most important aspect being the prompt correction of dehydration and acid-base and electrolyte disturbances. Paregoric or small doses of morphine may be used to relieve cramps and diarrhea, if contraindications do not exist, and in severe cases streptomycin or tetracycline may be of value. There is now some evidence, however, to suggest that the administration of antibiotics may prolong the carrier state (probably by upsetting intestinal ecology).

The control of salmonellosis is obviously a multidimensional situation. Certainly, everything possible must be done to detect and eliminate the infection at the animal source, and the state and federal authorities do a good job here considering the size of the problem. Further, meat, eggs, and milk must be protected by sanitary processing and stored foods should be safeguarded from possible contamination by flies and rodent feces. Patients should be isolated and carriers must be excluded from food handling until satisfactorily demonstrated to be "bacteriologically cured" (that is, no longer passing salmonellae). All of which means, of course, that food handlers and methods for preparing foods in public places must be under continuing supervision by local health departments.

Because most outbreaks involve inadequately cooked food, particularly poultry and eggs, the consumer's responsibility is clear enough. Unlike thermostable enterotoxin, salmonellae are killed easily at relatively moderate temperatures; for example, a few minutes exposure at 140°F. does the job. In actual practice, such temperatures must penetrate right to the center, and this is where the thermometer must reach in large roasts and birds. Occasionally, though, in spite of proper roasting, sufficient heat may not penetrate into the interior to destroy all salmonellae in the heavily contaminated large stuffed turkey. Again, the salmonellae in the yolk of the contaminated egg have been known to live through three-minute boiling, sunny-side up frying, and light scrambling.

Refrigeration is of obvious concern, too. The growth of bacteria is prevented when the *internal* temperature is at or below 42°F., and storage even at 50°F. may be safe for a few days if the food is not grossly contaminated. But higher temperatures are a different matter. For example, the salmonella count in experimentally contaminated ham salad remained at one million cells (per gram) at 42°F., but rose to 10 million in two days at 95°F.; and in experimentally contaminated chicken à la king it rose from one million to 100 million in two days at 95°F.! Refrigeration is especially critical in dealing with foods and dishes that are not cooked, such as the ham salad. Cool temperatures certainly do not eradicate salmonellae, but in mild contamination it may very well *prevent* a population explosion and consequent poisoning. . . . Prophylactically, anyway, salmonellosis boils down to this: "Cool to prevent" and "heat to kill."

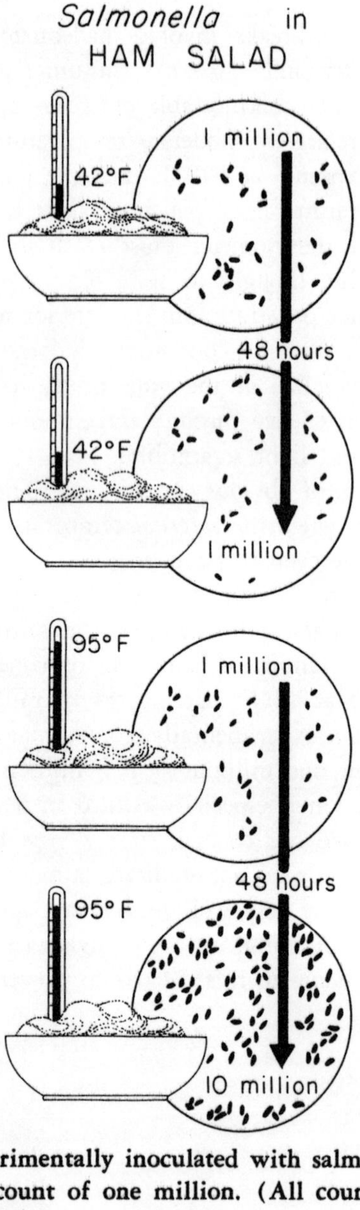

Ham salad experimentally inoculated with salmonellae, yielding a starting cell count of one million. (All counts refer to cells per gram of salad.)

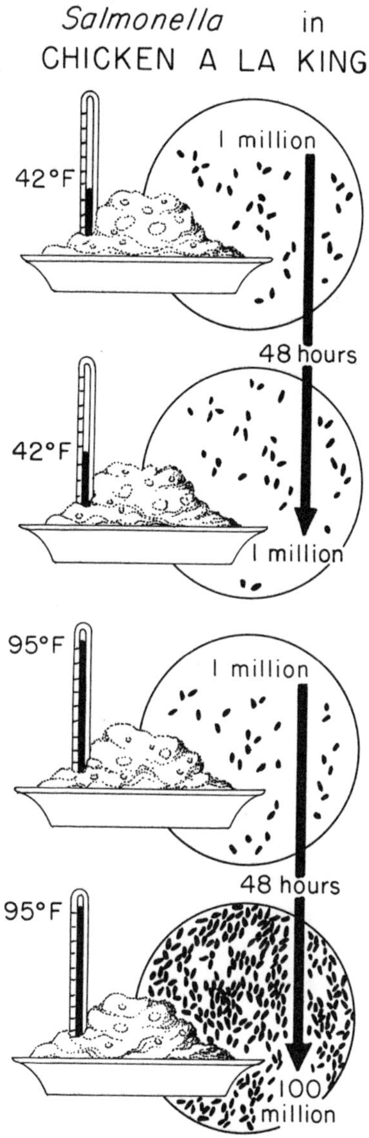

Chicken à la king inoculated experimentally with salmonellae, yielding a *starting* cell count of one million. (All counts refer to cells per gram of food.)

4
Roast Beef

In 1951 a new development appeared on the food poisoning scene, a mild gastroenteritis caused by *Clostridium perfringens* —a relative of the lethal *Clostridium botulinum.* The reason why the organism did not turn up before was that the routine culturing techniques in use (in "nonbotulism" outbreaks) did not exclude oxygen; clostridia—all clostridia—are anaerobes.

As a cause of gas gangrene, there was, paradoxically, nothing new about the species *Clostridium perfringens,* but much subsequent research has shown that the strain that causes food poisoning is not the same as the "gangrene organism." They look alike, of course, but differ physiologically. Above all, the food strain forms extremely heat-resistant spores—spores, like those of *Clostridium botulinum,* which resist boiling for hours! This plus their common occurrence easily explains the high incidence of the poisoning. Of the reported individuals involved in foodborne outbreaks in the United States for 1971, 28 percent (3,667 cases) were due to *Clostridium perfringens.* This was second only to staph food poisoning, with a figure of 38 percent. *Clostridium perfringens* has been isolated from a high proportion of raw meat samples, from animal feces, and from stools of healthy human beings.

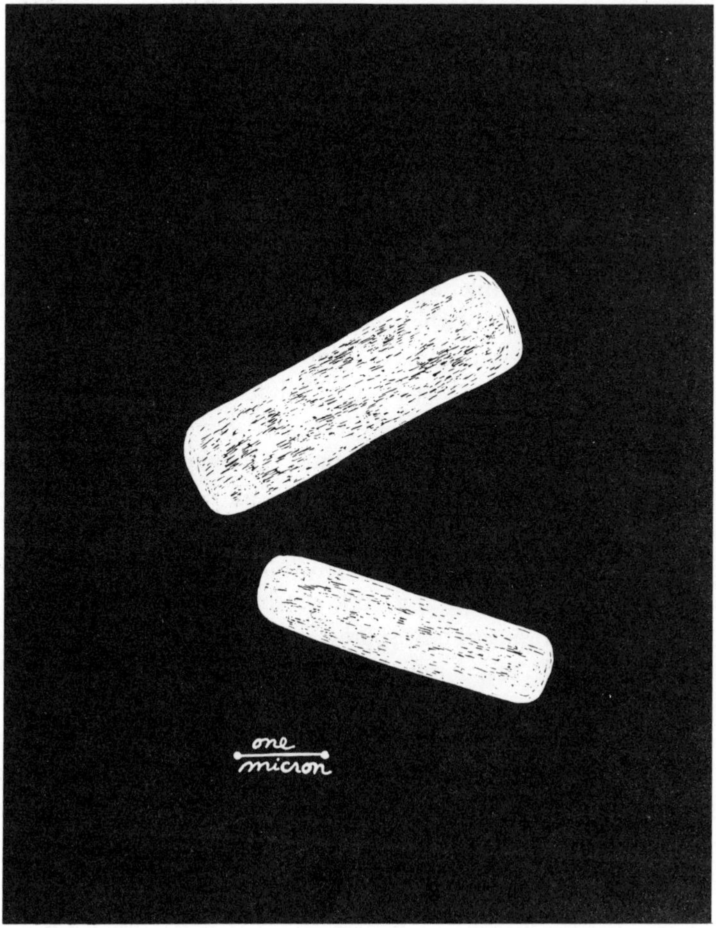

Clostridium perfringens, showing two bacilli. Although this is a spore-former, these particular cells are from a *young* culture and are without spores at this point.

Outbreaks frequently follow the eating of meat products that have been cooked and allowed to stand at warm temperatures. In such instances, the contaminating spores have not been destroyed and continue to grow when the product is not refrigerated. Beef (including gravy) is the most commonly incriminated food, followed by turkey and chicken (including dressing). Other "vehicles," to use the FDA expression, have included pork, fish, eggs, bakery products, fruits and vegetables, and Chinese food.

The mechanism of the illness caused by *Clostridium perfringens* is not completely understood, but presumably it is a matter of infection (of the intestinal mucosa) and consequent inflammation. The symptoms develop from within 8 to 24 hours after the meal and last just about 12 hours. Diarrhea is always present, usually accompanied by cramps, abdominal pain, and/or nausea. Vomiting is not common. Ordinarily, treatment is not indicated and there is almost always an uneventful recovery within 24 hours.

The diagnosis of an outbreak of *Clostridium perfringens* poisoning is made in the framework of the clinical situation and the isolation of anaerobic, spore-bearing bacilli from the incriminated food. The latter differ from *Clostridium botulinum* in several respects aside from their comparative benignity. They do not possess flagella (and therefore are not motile) but they do possess a capsule, or gelatinous covering. Unlike *Clostridium botulinum,* too, their spores are located more toward the center of the cell.

5
Dressing

Whereas staphylococci are cocci occurring in grapelike bunches, streptococci are cocci occurring in chains. Like staph, strep are ubiquitous and for the most part harmless. A drop of sour milk contains countless chains of *Streptococcus lactis,* the organism primarily responsible for sour cream, butter, buttermilk, and many cheeses. On the other hand, its look-alike cousin, *Streptococcus pyogenes,* is the cause of much sickness, including scarlet fever, rheumatic fever, strep throat, erysipelas, impetigo, cellulitis, and puerperal fever. And another troublemaker is *Streptococcus faecalis*—the cause of streptococcal food poisoning.

No one pretends to know the extent of strep food poisoning, but it may be considerable inasmuch as *Streptococcus faecalis* normally inhabits the intestines of both man and animals. This, of course, begs the question of why a "normal microbe" should incite illness. Presumably, the answer resides in the fact that in all outbreaks enormous numbers of the organism are ingested in the implicated food. Presumably, too, the mechanism by which illness results is a matter of infection rather than intoxication (as in the case of staph poisoning). That is, the strep invade and multiply within the intestinal lining to produce inflammation and associated signs and symptoms. There is, however, great variation in susceptibility among individuals. In one

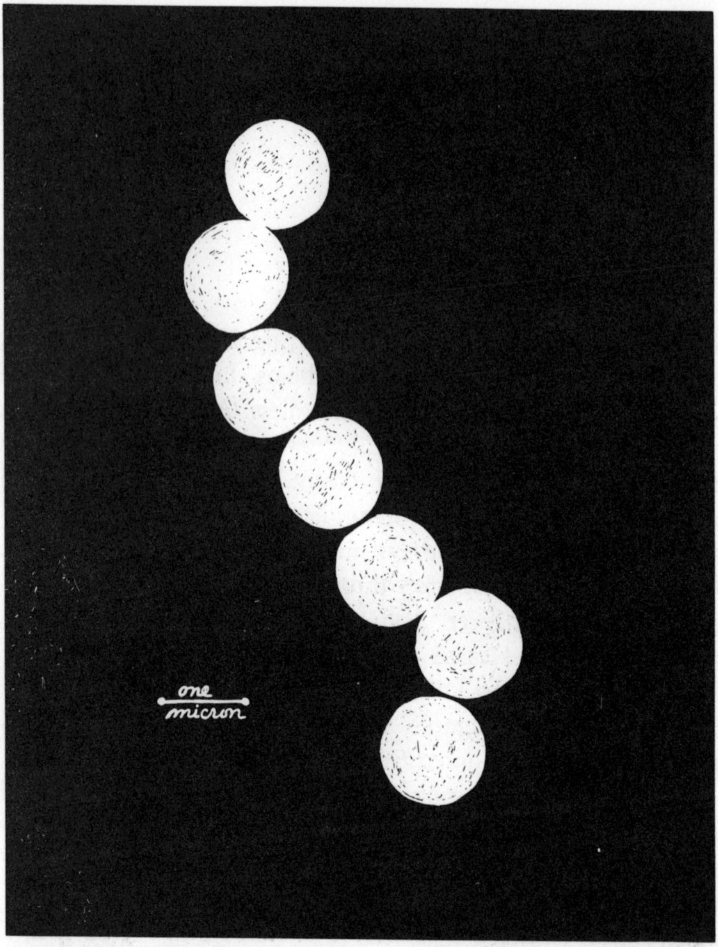

Streptococcus faecalis, the cause of streptococcal food poisoning. Shown is a single chain of seven cocci.

outbreak, for example, caused by turkey dressing at a banquet, 100 persons ate the poisoned food with impunity (293 became sick). Again, in an outbreak at a boys' school involving beef croquettes, *Streptococcus faecalis* felled 117 out of a total of 208. Further, in human volunteers illness often does not result even when large numbers of strep have been ingested in pure form. In sum, two factors operate in tandem just as in all food infections—"dose" (or number of organisms) and susceptibility. Accordingly, the pathological spectrum ranges from no sickness at all (low dose, low susceptibility), to pronounced poisoning (high dose, high susceptibility).

Strep food poisoning is much less severe than staph or salmonella poisoning, oftentimes amounting to no more than a "minor G.I. upset." Nevertheless, if reports of all such upsets were to filter into the offices of the Food and Drug Administration, strep poisoning could conceivably become a substantial statistic. Presently, it continues to command little attention and is *officially* responsible for only a small fraction of food poisonings. But a full-blown case of strep poisoning certainly commands the attention of its victims and for good reason—namely, nausea, cramps, and diarrhea (with occasional vomiting). The onset of symptoms usually varies from 2 to 18 hours after eating, with an average figure of some 12 hours. This is a much longer incubation period than staph poisonings and conforms to the idea that the involvement is basically a matter of microbial multiplication and inflammation. Symptoms almost always subside in the course of a few hours, and the treatment is entirely symptomatic.

Although the victim of an outbreak has recovered completely by the time the laboratory has arrived at the diagnosis, the latter nonetheless is an important step in the overall public health picture. In most instances the samples of the incriminated food are teeming with streptococci, and these are easily cultured, isolated, and identified. More particularly, when *Streptococcus faecalis* grows on blood agar its colonies are surrounded by a greenish halo (alpha hemolysis). Other strep produce colonies surrounded by a clear halo (beta hemolytic strep) or no halo at all (gamma strep). Actually, not all alpha hemolytic strep belong to the species *Streptococcus faecalis;* and for that matter not all strains of *Streptococcus faecalis* cause food poisoning. "Proof positive" necessitates the use of human volunteers, just as in staph poisoning. In the context of an outbreak with all the clinical earmarks of strep poisoning, however, the finding of alpha hemolytic streptococci in a food eaten by all victims is customarily taken to be a definitive diagnosis.

Outbreaks of strep food poisoning typically involve meat items, dressings, and the like, which have stood at room temperatures for a number of hours, allowing an explosive growth of *Streptococcus faecalis*. . . . Once again, *refrigerate!*

6
Pudding

Fairly similar in appearance to the clostridia is the species of bacteria by the name of *Bacillus cereus,* a relative newcomer to the family of microbes responsible for food poisoning—only but the very latest medical texts say anything at all about *Bacillus cereus* poisoning. Obviously, the bacterium is not new. What is new concerns the fact that it causes trouble under certain circumstances. Not much trouble, fortunately, yet enough to enlist the interest of the Food and Drug Administration.

Bacillus cereus is a common soil inhabitant; some strains are marked by the ability to form very long chains of cells. Unlike clostridia the microbe needs oxygen to grow and multiply, but like clostridia it is gram positive and forms highly *resistant* spores under adverse environmental conditions. If these spores happen to contaminate food and the temperature is "just right" —no refrigeration!—they burst forth into their active stage and multiply in a most vigorous way. And with sufficient time, the count will be high enough to set off an infectional gastroenteritis. Once again, the microbe per se is only half at fault—the cook does the rest.

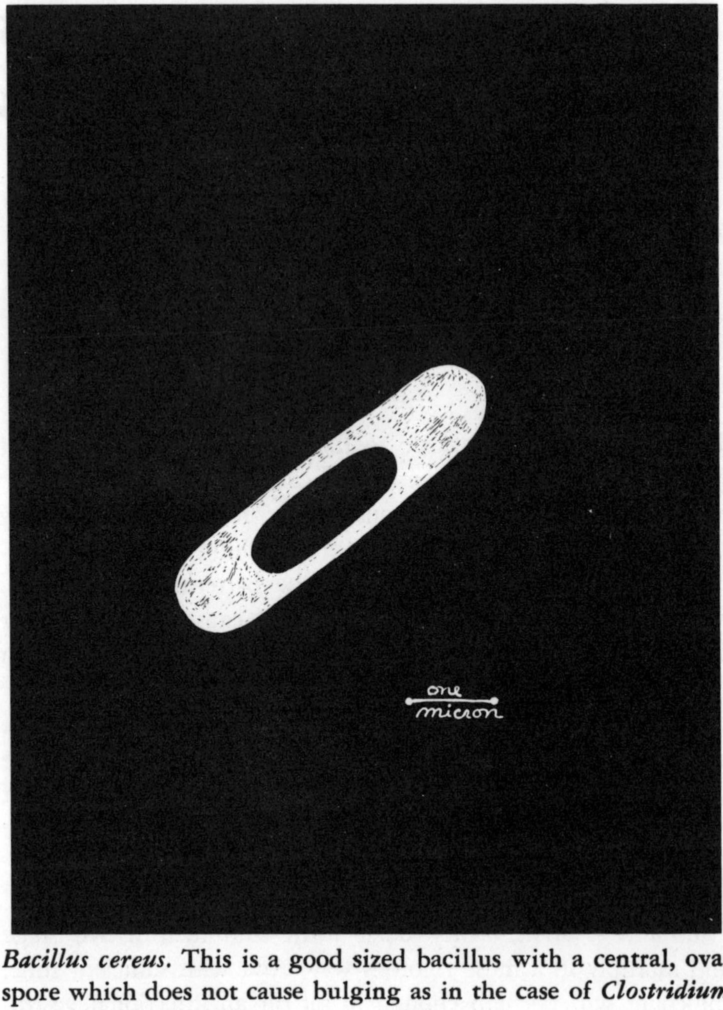

Bacillus cereus. This is a good sized bacillus with a central, oval spore which does not cause bulging as in the case of *Clostridium botulinum* (p. 21).

The inflammation produces the usual nausea, colicky pains, and diarrhea; occasionally there is vomiting. The incubation period runs around 6 hours, and the illness proper rarely lasts longer than 12 hours. All in all the involvement is relatively mild (clinically indistinguishable from *Clostridium perfringens* poisoning) and no therapy is indicated.

Bacillus cereus seems to do best in starchy foods, puddings, pastries and the like, although very few items fail to support the organism given an unrefrigerated situation and enough time. Recent outbreaks investigated by the FDA turned up bread pudding, doughnuts, gravy and, rather unexpectedly, oysters.

7
Salad

Shigellosis, or bacillary dysentery, is a severe gastroenteritis marked by frequent passage of stools (containing blood, pus, and mucus), abdominal cramps, malaise, and fever. Dehydration and circulatory collapse may lead to death, especially in debilitated adults and infants. The involvement is often indistinguishable from salmonellosis, which means, of course, that the offending agent must be isolated from the stools to establish the diagnosis. The classical mode of transmission is person-to-person contact via the fecal-oral route, thus explaining why many medical texts do not look upon shigellosis as food poisoning. There are enough outbreaks involving food, however, to justify a few remarks in a book of this sort. In 1971, for instance, the Center for Disease Control reported 1,040 cases through their food-borne surveillance system. Considering that few outbreaks are reported to the proper authorities, the actual figure is undoubtedly much higher than this. The foods associated with shigellosis outbreaks have included beef, turkey, fruits, vegetables, salads, and poi. The 1970 "poi outbreak" in Hawaii involved over a thousand cases.

The "offending agents" of shigellosis are rod-shaped bacteria

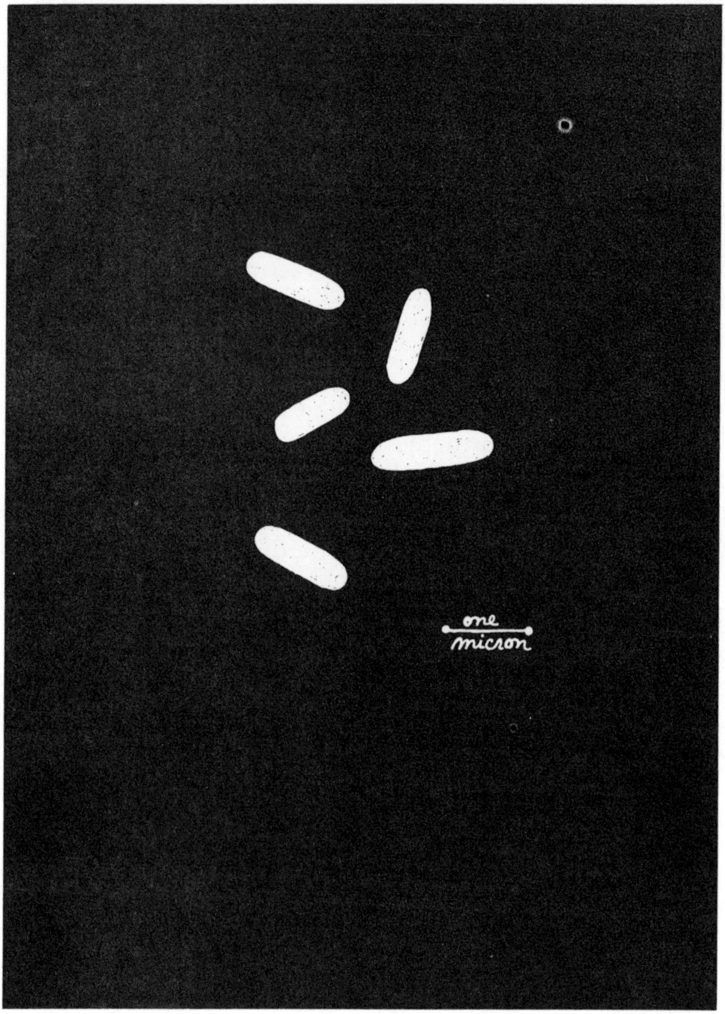

Shigella dysenteriae, a major cause of shigellosis. Five bacilli (cells) are shown. Except for their lack of flagella shigellae are indistinguishable from salmonellae (p. 50).

(bacilli) called shigellae (in honor of the Japanese bacteriologist, Kiyoshi Shiga). Except for their lack of flagella and motility, shigellae easily pass for salmonellae. Also remindful of salmonellae, there are dozens of species and countless types. The major pathogens, *Shigella flexneri, Shigella sonnei, Shigella boydii,* and *Shigella dysenteriae,* look alike, exactly alike, and it takes sophisticated laboratory procedures to tell which is which. Once ingested, however, there may be considerable difference in the ensuing infection, *Shigella dysenteriae* being particularly virulent. For epidemiological purposes, especially, it is most important to determine the precise species and type in a given outbreak.

The incubation period varies from one to four days. In infants and small children the onset is sudden and explosive—nausea, vomiting, diarrhea, abdominal pain and distention, and fever. Typically, the stools become bloody and increase to 20 or more a day. Dehydration is severe. In the adult the situation is essentially the same save for the fever and bloody stools. Mild infections last about a week, and severe infections may extend to a couple of months. Treatment centers on the use of intravenous fluids to combat dehydration and to replace lost salt and other vital minerals. In most cases antibiotics are not needed, but they are commonly given to shorten the duration of the diarrhea and to prevent the patient from becoming a carrier.

The control of shigellosis includes isolation during the acute stage and disinfection of feces and all contaminated articles. Good sanitation and hygiene are musts and carriers should not handle or prepare food. Interestingly, foods and dishes that necessitate considerable handling and preparation are well-recognized vehicles. Potato salad is the classic example.

8
Clams

Early on the morning of September 14, 1972, a Patrol Warden attached to the Parker Wildlife Reservation at Plum Island (Massachusetts) reported an extensive bird kill (ducks and gulls) at the Merrimack River estuary. And before noon on the same day a *reddish brown* mass of marine growth was reported at Hodgkins Cove, twelve miles south. In a matter of hours scientists at the University of Massachusetts Marine Biological Laboratory identified the growth as the microscopic and highly dangerous *Gonyaulax tamarensis.* And one quart of sea water was found to contain sufficient cells to kill a mouse in a few minutes' time. At 2 P.M.—still on the same day—the Massachusetts Department of Public Health declared the North Shore region from Gloucester to the New Hampshire line closed to the taking of shellfish, and the following day, September 15, Governor Francis W. Sargent declared a public health emergency. As a control measure, an immediate embargo was placed upon the sale and marketing of fresh and frozen shellfish at the wholesale and retail levels. By the 16th the harvesting of all shellfish along the Massachusetts coastline was banned and the control program extended to include the confiscation of all shelf-stock in markets and restaurants; further, a total import and export embargo was enforced. Meanwhile, the press, radio, and television spread the alarm—Red Tide!—and hospitals and physicians throughout the state were informed of the signs and symptoms of the poisoning and the recommended treatment. Considering the fact that thousands of acres of shellfish harvesting areas were found to be contaminated, the Health Department's speedy action quite possibly saved dozens of lives. Certainly it stemmed an epidemic. As it was there were only 26 reported and confirmed cases of shellfish poisoning.

The Red Tide could very well be one of man's oldest *recognized* epidemics. Ancient writings often speak of it and in none other than Exodus (7:20–21) we read ". . . And all the waters that were in the river turned to blood. And the fish that were in them died." What was clearly shellfish poisoning was well-documented in France in 1689, and in our own history the first "outbreak" occurred in 1903 at Timber Cove, California. The first *major* outbreak occurred in 1926 in the San Francisco area with 102 cases of poisoning and 6 deaths. In Canada outbreaks have occurred in 1936 in Nova Scotia, in 1945 on both the New Brunswick and Nova Scotia sides of the Bay of Fundy, and sporadically to the present time. The causative organism on the West Coast has been identified as *Gonyaulax catenella,* and on the East Coast as the species already mentioned—*Gonyaulax tamarensis.*

The various species of *Gonyaulax* belong to a large group of microscopic marine algae called dinoflagellates. All possess flagella (whiplike propellers) and all tend to be brownish in color. Specifically, *Gonyaulax tamarensis* is roundish (some 35 microns in diameter) and moves by means of two flagella. The generation time for this species and other dinoflagellates relates to temperature, light intensity, salinity, and nutrient concentration. Calm seas, low concentrations of nitrogen and phosphorus,

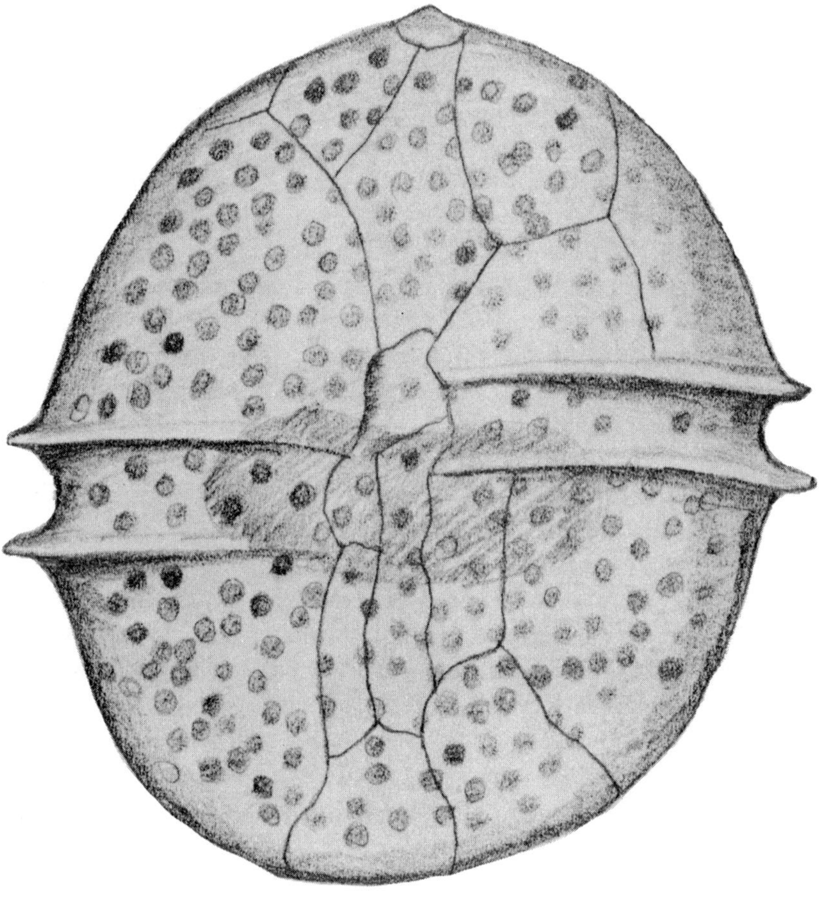

The marine dinoflagellate *Gonyaulax tamarensis.*

and a surface temperature of about 50°F. are *some* of the factors that stimulate growth and provoke Red Tides.

The tasteless toxin synthesized by marine dinoflagellates is 50 times stronger than curare, the arrow poison used by some South American Indians. What is more, mussels, clams, oysters, and other filter-feeding shellfish ingest vast numbers of such organisms and concentrate the poison in their livers. Often referred to as mytilotoxin (from the Greek *mytilos*—mussel), as little as 125 micrograms may produce severe poisoning in man and 500 micrograms (1/60,000 ounce!) has proved fatal. Whereas the international standard for shellfish considers any value greater than 80 micrograms per 100 grams of meat to be hazardous, the contaminated Massachusetts clams registered some 4,000 micrograms. Translated to the dinner table, this meant that three such clams contained a lethal dose!

The first symptoms of paralytic shellfish poisoning (PSP), to use the expression of the Massachusetts Department of Public Health (or mussel poisoning, or mytilotoxism in deference to other sources), generally commence within a half hour following the meal. These include numbness and tingling of the lips, face and tongue and prickling of the fingers and toes. Also, some victims experience a peculiar feeling of lightness and a floating or flying sensation. Later on, there is muscle weakness gradually progressing to the neck, arms, and legs which eventually may lead to complete paralysis of the extremities. In fatal cases, death results in 3 to 12 hours from respiratory failure. Victims who survive the first 12 hours usually recover rapidly without lingering effects. Because there is no specific antidote treatment is primarily symptomatic, consisting of the evacuation of the poison from the body via vomiting, gastric lavage and catharsis, and combating breathing difficulties through the use of artificial respiration and oxygen.

Part Two
NONMICROBIAL POISONING

9 Fish

Contrary to what instinct and intuition seem to tell us, not all fish are edible and, what is more, some are extremely poisonous. About 15,000 species of fish are recognized, and somewhere in the neighborhood of 300 or so have been reported to cause intoxication or, as the medical dictionary puts it, icthyosarcotoxism (for our purpose, fish poisoning). And for the sake of explicitness, we are not talking about bites or stings or bacterial contamination or allergic reactions, but rather the toxic effects arising from the eating of the flesh, liver, or roe. The incidence of poisoning may be as high as 5 to 50 percent of the population in tropical countries where fish forms a large part of the diet. About 100 cases are reported yearly in Hawaii, and in Japan the death toll is some 100 each year.

With one or two exceptions, the toxins at the root of fish poisoning are shrouded in chemical mystery. Further, there is no way of telling for sure whether these poisonings are "inherent" or acquired by feeding on poisonous plankton (fish food). For the most part the latter idea appears the more useful because of the well-recognized influences of season and geography. The surgeonfish, the filefish, the goatfish, and the porcupine fish, to cite a few examples, are poisonous only a part of the year in the same localities. Still other fish, including the barracuda, pompano, mackerel, snapper, sea bass, perch, and wrasse are sporadically poisonous in certain localities and in other places are always safe to eat. In contrast, though, are those species that are dangerous at most any time and thus appear to be "born that way." These include fish of the Tetraodontidae family, and most especially, the balloon fish, globefish, toadfish, and puffers. Poisoning by such fish (tetraodontoxism) is severe and commonly deadly, with an overall mortality rate close to 75 percent.

Comparatively little is known, as noted, about the chemistry and mechanism of action of the toxins of poisonous fish and merely for convenience are they dubbed "icthyosarcotoxins." In regard to puffers, however, a potent toxin, called tetraodontoxin, has been isolated and chemically identified. Secreted in the ovaries of the fish and present also in high concentrations in the liver, tetraodontoxin attacks the nerve endings of its victim and in lethal amounts causes death by respiratory paralysis. About a half milligram—a mere speck—is deadly! All in all it acts very much like mytilotoxin of poisonous *shellfish,* and the same more or less applies to the toxins present in other poisonous fish.

The signs and symptoms of fish poisoning develop within a very short time, almost always within an hour of ingestion, and run the gamut of toxicologic dishevelment. First, and typically, there is numbness and tingling of the face and lips which spreads to the fingers and toes, later followed by nausea, vomiting, diarrhea, malaise, dizziness, abdominal pain, chills, fever, sweating, painful urination, numbness of the limbs, incoordination and muscular weakness. In the severe case there is foaming at the mouth, labored breathing, paralysis, and convulsions; death may occur from respiratory failure within a matter of hours. There is great variation, of course; a given poisoning

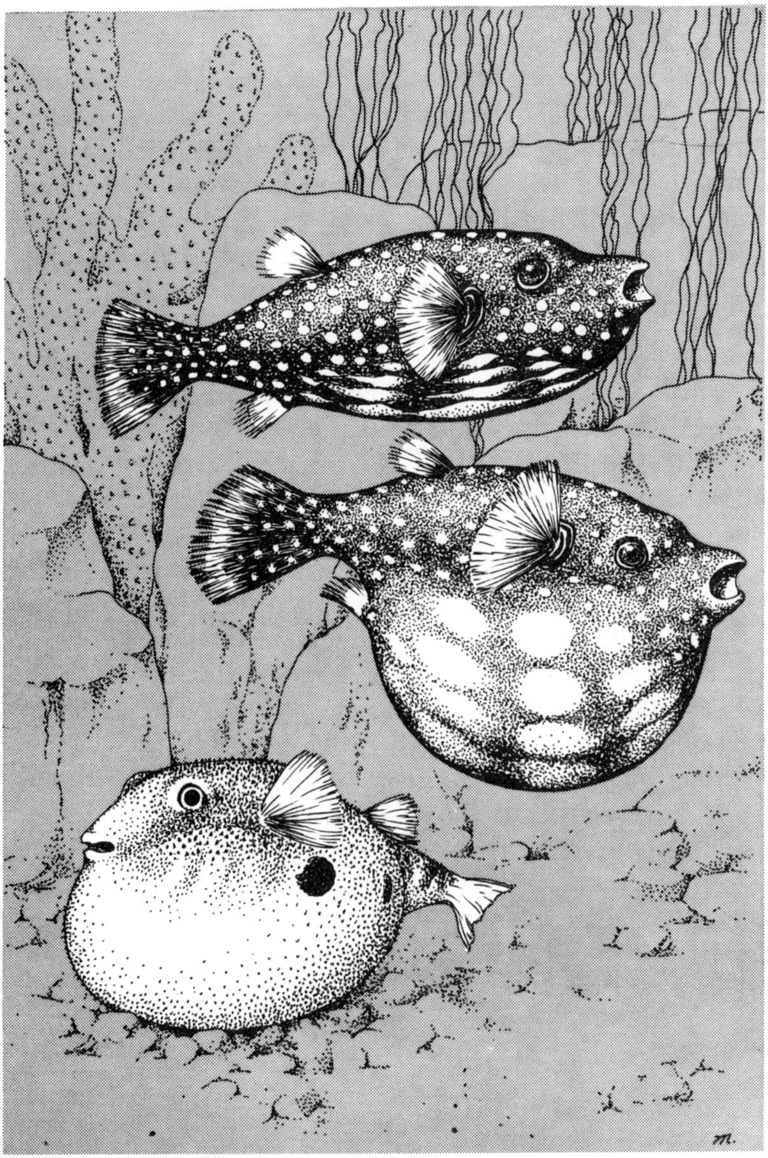

Typical puffer or blowfish. (In actual practice these terms refer to various marine fishes of the family Tetraodontidae that are capable of swelling up.)

actually represents an interplay of the amount of toxin ingested, the kind of fish, and the victim's physiological makeup. Among those who recover, and most do unless a tetraodont is involved, muscular weakness and perverted sensations of the face, lips, and mouth may wear on for weeks.

Treatment centers on the removal of ingested fish (via induced vomiting, gastric lavage, and catharsis) and proper management of convulsions and paralysis. Not surprisingly, there is no specific antidote, but a dozen hours or so of artificial respiration may be lifesaving. The prognosis in any particular outbreak is difficult to predict since mortality varies anywhere from less than 1 percent to more than 70 percent. As a rule of thumb, however, the lower rate may be expected when the fish is known to be a common type and normally edible.

In tropical countries the prevention of fish poisoning is clearly of paramount importance in the public health program. Many species are never safe to eat and many, too, are not safe to eat at certain times of year or in certain localities. Actually, it demands the talents of the expert, more so even than mushrooming. Japan has strict laws in this area, particularly when it comes to the gastronomic sport of eating fugu, a highly toxic globefish with delicate and delicious white flesh. In restaurants specially licensed to serve this potentially dangerous food, the chef must pass a stringent examination to test his knowledge of the fish species, the seasonal variation, and cunning skills of eviscerating the fish without contaminating the flesh.

10 Mushrooms

Fungi are lowly plants without chlorophyll. They include yeasts, molds, mildews, rusts, smuts, puffballs, and, central to our interest here, mushrooms and toadstools. *Webster's Third New International Dictionary* gives first-place status to the view that toadstools are umbrella-shaped fungi ("period"), while the *American Heritage Dictionary of the English Language* defines the word as "an inedible fungus with an umbrella-shaped fruiting body, as distinguished from an edible mushroom." The latter agrees with Webster's *second* entry, to wit: "A fleshy fungus that is poisonous or inedible as distinguished from an edible mushroom." Interestingly, modern usage eschews toadstool, the fairyland hallmark usually giving way to "poisonous mushroom."

Mushrooms, in actual practice, run the gamut from items of gastronomic elegance to deadly poisons, with "suspect," "nonedible," and species of "little interest" occupying a vast botanical twilight zone. In Europe, where mushrooming is widely practiced, poisoning is far from uncommon, and even here at home there are about 100 fatalities each year. Practically all of these deaths relate to the species *Amanita phalloides,* which, among others, is popularly called "death cap," "death cup," "deadly amanita," and "green death cap." Second runner-up (a poor second) is *Amanita muscaria* ("fly agaric" or "muscaria"). Occasionally, poisoning occurs from the eating of *Amanita verna* ("destroying angel"), which is just as poisonous as death cap but not nearly as common, and the much less dangerous *Gyromitra esculenta* ("false morel"). In Europe, *Amanita pantherina* ("false blushes") is responsible for a fair number of poisonings and deaths. And as Nature is wont to operate, the bad *Amanitae* are balanced by the good *Amanitae—Amanita caesarea* and *Amanita rubescens* ("blusher") being highly esteemed mushrooms.

The poisonous principle of *Amanita phalloides* and *Amanita verna* was isolated in crystalline form by Lynen and Wieland (1937) and appropriately named phalloidin. It is present in both the cap and stem in high concentrations and a mere taste of the mushroom may cause serious poisoning; a good bite may cause death! Phalloidin is toxic to all cells, and it is especially injurious to the liver, kidney, brain, and heart. The first signs and symptoms usually appear in 6 to 16 hours "after the meal," though in some cases not before a day or two. These include nausea, vomiting, diarrhea, stomach pains, headache, mental confusion, cold sweat, irregular heart, and labored breathing. Later the liver becomes hard and swollen, the blood pressure falls, the skin yellows, and coma ensues. In fatal cases death occurs in five to ten days; in nonfatal cases the victim recovers gradually but aftereffects remain for a long time, sometimes for life. Other things being equal the chances for survival are about fifty-fifty; or, as one text puts it, "the prognosis of poisoning from *Amanita phalloides* is bad."

Although most works and handbooks on poisoning stress the removal of the toxic material by emesis, catharsis, and washing out the stomach (gastric lavage), the *Merck Manual* notes that little is gained through such measures if there has been

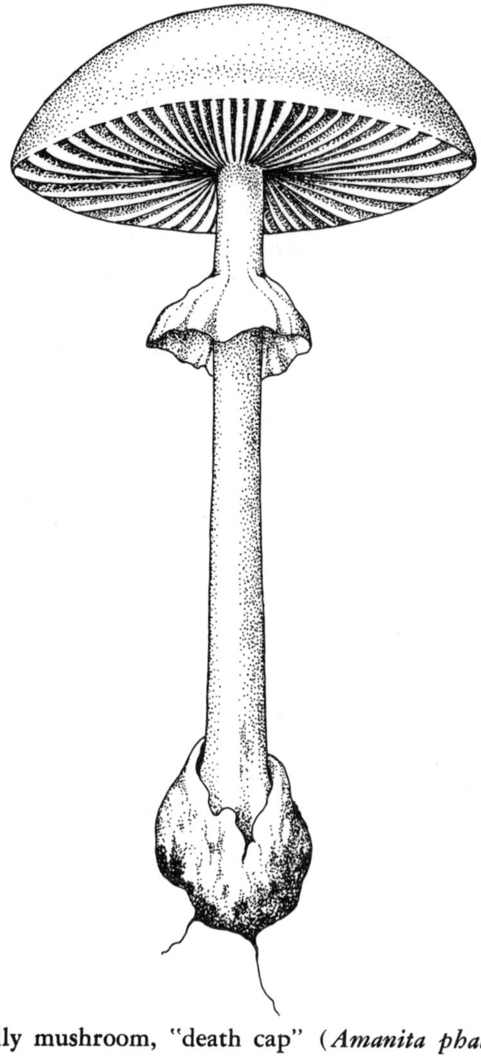

The deadly mushroom, "death cap" (*Amanita phalloides*).

violent vomiting or diarrhea, or if the symptoms appear several hours later. Otherwise, of course, they are the first object in treatment in order to stem further absorption of phalloidin. More general measures include absolute bed rest, intravenous fluids to check dehydration and shock, and analgesics for pain. Also, a high-carbohydrate diet supplemented by intravenous dextrose is considered of value in helping to prevent liver damage.

The chief poison in *Amanita muscaria* is muscarine, a powerful stimulant of certain nerves supplying the vital organs. The toxic effects, which begin within a few minutes to two hours after eating the mushroom, include salivation, sweating, tearing, nausea, vomiting, retching, thirst, colic, mucous and bloody stools, labored breathing, cold, clammy skin, uncontrollable urination, and staggering gait. Not uncommonly, there are giddiness and mental confusion, excitability, shrieking, dancing up and down, and even fits of raving madness. Collapse and coma, and occasionally convulsions, supervene in severe poisoning, and in fatal cases death results from respiratory failure or cardiac arrest. But other things being equal, the prognosis is good; most victims are back to normal again in a day or two.

Treatment of *Amanita muscaria* poisoning centers on the evacuation of ingested mushrooms by induced vomiting and gastric lavage, and the giving of atropine to antagonize the action of muscarine. For example, whereas the latter slows the heart, atropine speeds the heart. In the management of cases marked by exceptional excitement, however, atropine must be used with caution, because it itself is somewhat of a cerebral stimulant. Other important measures are bed rest and the giving of intravenous fluids and sedatives.

The answer to mushroom poisoning is actually a matter of scientific common sense. Above all, there are no general rules or empirical means of distinguishing the good from the bad.

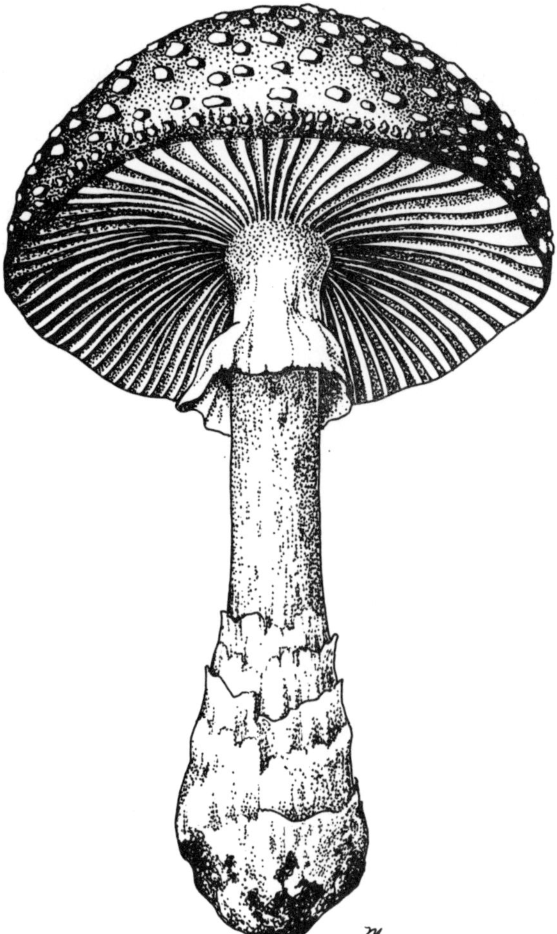

The poison mushroom, "fly agaric" (*Amanita muscaria*).

Poisonous mushrooms *do not* taste bitter (death cap is almost *tasteless!*); they *do not* turn yellow when salted; they *do not* turn silver black; they *do not* turn blue when cut; and so on. The good and the bad can be distinguished only on a basis of botanical characteristics, and this demands the talents of the expert. And the only way to become an expert is to mushroom for years and years under the watchful eye of an expert teacher, preferably an octogenarian who has picked and eaten mushrooms all his life and is alive to tell about it. Without such tutelage the only wise course is to be satisfied with cultivated mushrooms. They are good—and safe!

11
Fava Beans

That morning the boy (age five) felt fine, but by early afternoon he complained of stomach pains and vomited. He was very pale, had a headache and temperature, and passed reddish (wine-colored) urine. The cramps continued throughout the night, and the next morning the skin was yellow and became much more so as the day wore on; the cramps still continued and there was frequent yawning. In late afternoon he was admitted to the hospital with all the foregoing signs and symptoms plus the laboratory findings of a red cell count of 1.5 million (normal, 4 to 5 million!) and a white cell count of 33,000 (normal, 7–10,000!). A pint of blood was given immediately to correct the anemia and this did indeed bring about the desired effect. Other than the temperature remaining up until the fourth day, recovery proved, as the doctors say, "uneventful."

The diagnosis came into full bloom in the framework of the boy's history. To wit, the day before the onset of illness his grandmother had cooked a quantity of fava beans, of which he had eaten "four plates full." Moreover, two years before, at the age of three, there was a similar episode following such a meal. That bout lasted for two weeks, but then cleared up spontaneously without treatment. Further, the boy was Italian! In other words, fava beans plus the Mediterranean basin spells biochemical trouble or, as the medical dictionary puts it, favism. More precisely, a fair percentage of the peoples of the basin harbor a defective gene which remains in the family, a gene responsible for the *lack* of an essential red cell enzyme dubbed "G6PD." Such red cells are easily destroyed by stressful situations, including certain chemicals, drugs, *and fava beans.* That is, they burst apart (hemolysis) and thereby release and lose their oxygen carrying hemoglobin. The upshot is hemolytic anemia and its various manifestations. Of special note, the liberated hemoglobin colors the urine red and its breakdown products color the skin yellow (jaundice).

Interestingly, not all G6PD-deficient persons are prone to favism. This suggests the involvement of additional defective genes and the necessity of inheriting all of them together in order to yield red cells sufficiently defective to result in favism. And as to the exact chemical constituent of the bean triggering the hemolysis there is no unanimous opinion. Several agents have been singled out, including L-Dopa, perhaps the most effective drug ever discovered to control certain forms of Parkinson's disease. Indeed, fava beans are the commercial source!

Fava or fava bean (also faba) is the specific epithet of the broad bean *Vicia fava,* a staple item of the diet in Italy, Sicily, and Sardinia. Actually, it is fairly common throughout the Mediterranean basin, and so is favism. Here at home the bean is grown in several states and a fair amount is imported from Italy as canned food. Accordingly, favism is not exactly rare; or at the very least it is something to be considered when the doctor encounters a sudden case of hemolytic anemia. Further, susceptible persons may contract favism just by inhaling the

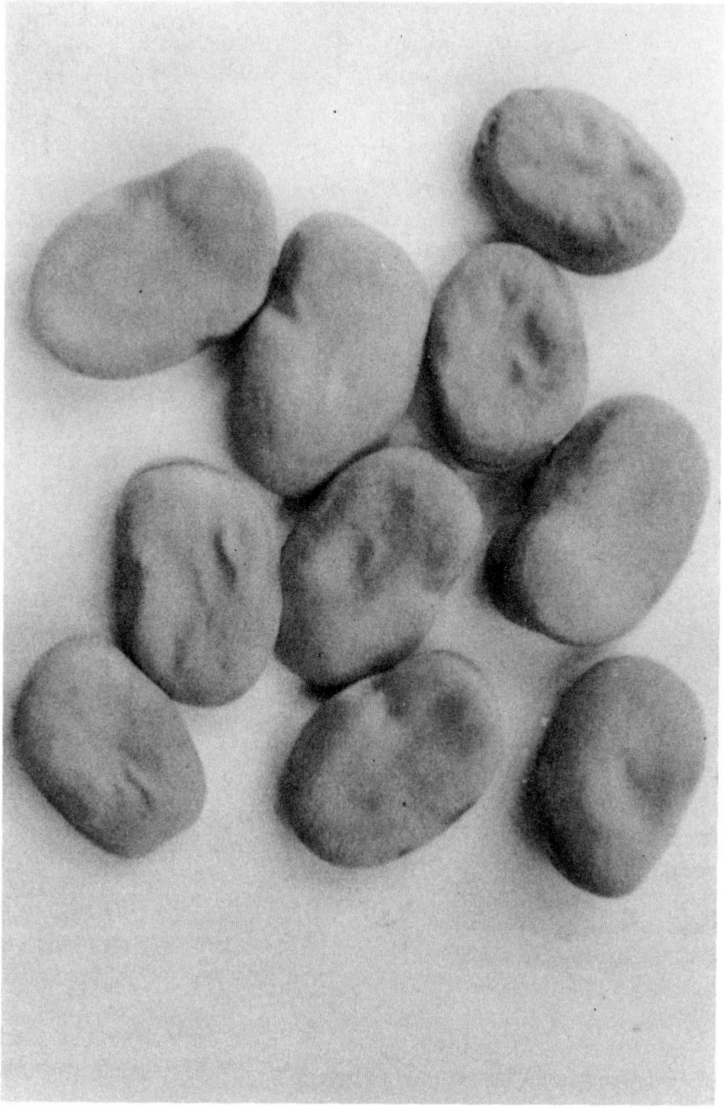

Fava beans (*Vicia fava*).

pollen, and this especially must be kept in mind in those localities where the plant is extensively cultivated.

The onset of poisoning varies from minutes to a day or so and the usual attack lasts about five days. The severe case may run for several weeks! Typical features include malaise, vomiting, diarrhea, dizziness, abdominal pain, elevated temperature, headache, yawning, marked pallor, jaundice, red to black urine, enlarged liver, and often loss of consciousness. And at the test-tube level, the red cell count is way down and the white cell count way up. Blood transfusions effect good results and death is rare except in children. Known susceptibles most certainly should avoid fava beans, and none other than Pythagoras, who reputedly suffered from favism, counseled "never to walk in bean fields."

12
Milk

Daniel Boone and his followers had much to contend with, not the least of which was an attractive weed by the name of white snakeroot (botanically, *Eupatorium urticoefolium*). Clearly, its roots did not cure snakebite, but the plant did indeed poison and kill cattle—and did indeed poison the milk. Cattle got the "trembles" (trembling is uniformly seen) and humans suffered "milk sickness." There is every reason to believe that milk sickness killed Lincoln's mother, just as it did untold thousands of other settlers throughout the Midwest.

White snakeroot grows abundantly in heavily wooded areas, and this is where cattle head when grazing is scarce—and when *free* to do so. Trembles and milk sickness still occasionally pop up, particularly in the midwestern and southwestern parts of the country. In the Southwest, though, the troublemaker is not usually snakeroot, but a close relative called jimmy weed or rayless goldenrod (*Aplopappus heterophyllus*). Both plants contain high concentrations of an aromatic, straw-colored alcohol aptly termed tremetol, first isolated (and proved to be the toxic principle) in 1917 at the laboratories of the United States Department of Agriculture.

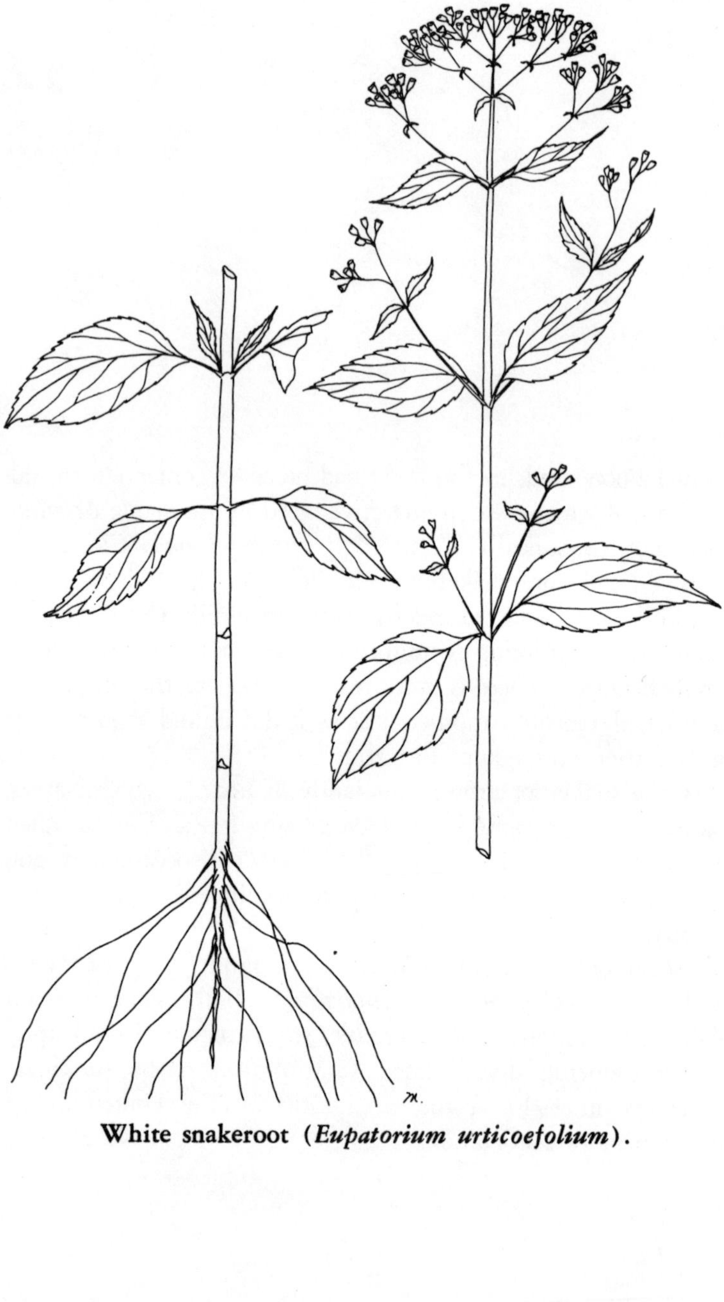

White snakeroot (*Eupatorium urticoefolium*).

The mechanism of tremetol poisoning is not well understood, except for the very definite damage to the pancreas, liver, and kidney noted at autopsy. The signs and symptoms commence a few hours following ingestion and include just about every wayward physiological event imaginable. Weakness, prostration, severe vomiting, abdominal pain, flushed cheeks, red tongue and lips, great thirst, and a falling temperature and blood pressure are prominent features. Also, acetone appears in the blood (as a result of acidosis) and eventually gives the breath a faint odor remindful of nailpolish remover. The uncontrolled diabetic exhales acetone, too, but in stark contrast to that disease tremetol *reduces* blood sugar. On the other hand it shoots up blood waste products, presumably because of its toxic effects upon the kidney. In fatal cases, death is preceded by convulsions and coma, and in victims who recover weakness persists for days, weeks, or even months, depending on the severity of the attack.

The diagnosis of milk sickness is usually not a problem in light of the characteristic signs and symptoms and the fact that several cases appear pretty much at once. Further, a blood test will show acetone and low blood sugar, and, to boot, tremetol can be chemically tested for in the milk. Regarding treatment, there is no known antidote against tremetol, which means that the doctor can do no more than control the symptoms. Bed rest is essential, and a high-carbohydrate diet (plus B-complex vitamins) is generally believed to protect the liver. Other helpful measures are the giving of baking soda to combat the acidosis and the use of the artificial kidney in the event of renal failure. The old mountaineers traditionally treated milk sickness with whiskey and honey, but there is excellent reason for eschewing alcohol in light of what we know about the kidney and liver. The honey makes sense, of course. . . . Best of all, keep the cows away from snakeroot and jimmy weed. (Unfortunately, pasteurization does not destroy tremetol.)

13
Potatoes

Few families of the plant kingdom are more interesting or valuable than the one by the name of *Solanaceae.* To this great family of some 2,000 species belong scores of important medicinal plants, tobacco, eggplant, the tomato, and the potato. Not surprisingly, these plants look alike and harbor many of the same chemical compounds, some of which are potent—and dangerous!—drugs. Belladonna, or deadly nightshade, for example, yields the much-used medicinals atropine and scopolamine. Both drugs act upon the peripheral nervous system to produce similar effects; both act upon the brain, but in "opposite directions." Atropine stimulates and in toxic doses causes convulsions, whereas scopolamine depresses and in toxic doses brings on a deep sleep and loss of consciousness. In therapeutic doses, scopolamine is somewhat of a tranquilizer and truth serum, and years ago was used along with morphine to produce "twilight sleep" in childbirth—a state in which the patient, while responding to pain, does not retain it in her memory.

Not to be pharmacologically outdone, the potato, too, contains a few "active principles," and most especially a poison called solanine (after the plant's botanical name, *Solanum tuberosum*). Solanine is contained in all green parts and particularly in the berrylike fruits. The eating of just a few of these berries

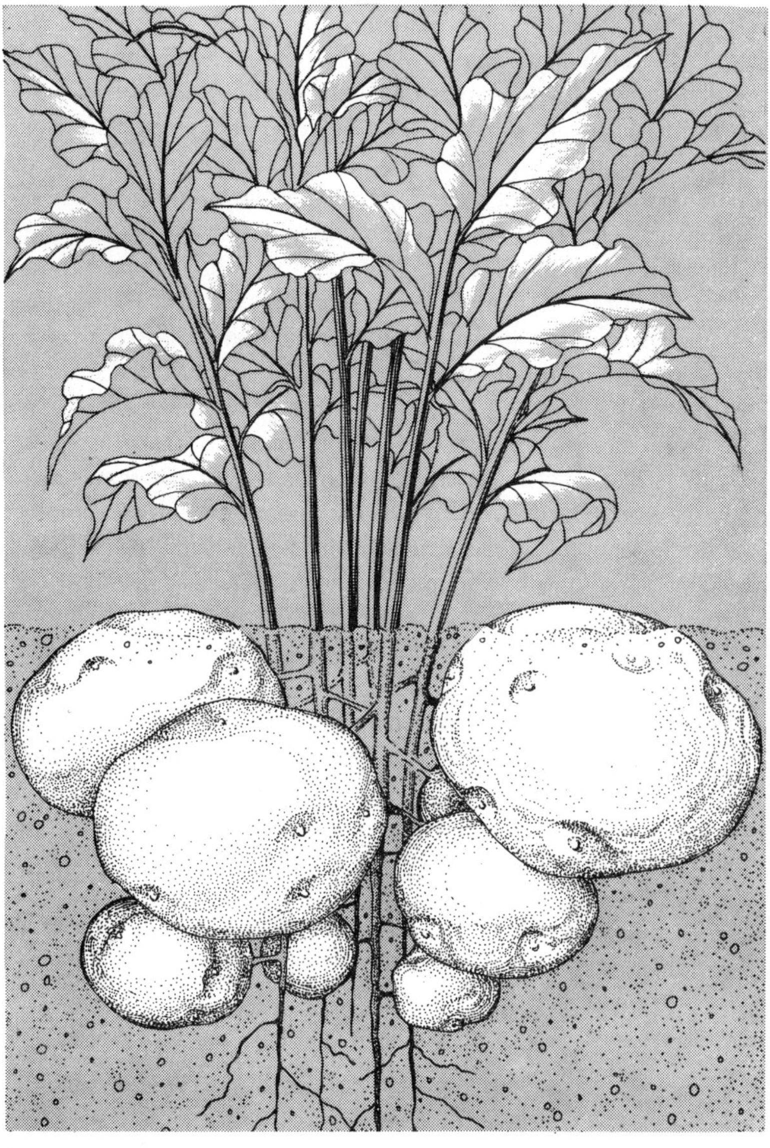

The potato (*Solanum tuberosum*).

can cause severe poisoning and even death. Mature potato tubers—the potato we eat—contain insignificant amounts of solanine but *immature* (green) and vigorously sprouting potatoes may contain toxic but rarely lethal amounts. The signs and symptoms of potato poisoning occur within a few hours and consist of nausea, vomiting, diarrhea, abdominal pain, headache, anxiety, cold and clammy skin, weakness, dizziness, dilated pupils, a sense of constriction in the throat, and prostration. In some cases the liver is enlarged, and the patient may hemorrhage and collapse. Other than the removal of the poison via induced vomiting, gastric lavage, and catharsis, the management amounts to the control of symptoms as they arise.

Very closely allied to potato poisoning is that caused by "bittersweet," both species of which belong to the same genus as the potato. *Solanum dulcamara,* commonly known as European bittersweet, blue nightshade, and woody nightshade, is a woody climbing or reclining herb with slender stems and dark, pointed leaves that may be purplish-green when young. Clusters of white or purplish-white flowers give rise to attractive bright red berries well charged with solanine. *Solanum nigrum* (American bittersweet, black nightshade, or poison berry) closely resembles European bittersweet, except for having purple or black berries. These too contain solanine. Both bittersweets occur in numerous areas (generally in moist, rich soil conditions) and are the bane of the unwary berry picker. The signs and symptoms and treatment are the same as for potato poisoning.

14
Rye Bread

When migraine strikes, the only remedy known to afford real relief is a drug by the name of ergotamine; when bleeding continues in the wake of childbirth the best remedy is ergonovine. Both of these drugs, as their name suggests, hail from the same source, and a rather unlikely source at that; they are found in a lowly fungus called ergot, and most especially the species (*Claviceps purpurea*) which attacks rye and related grains. Not surprisingly, therefore, the ingestion of ergot-contaminated flour—bread!—provides unwanted doses of ergotamine and ergonovine and causes ergot poisoning. In the past ergotism was not uncommon and occurred in epidemic form, but today, thanks to modern methods, it occurs only sporadically and, in the United States, almost not at all.

What happens in ergotism interestingly relates to the therapeutic uses of ergotamine and ergonovine. Supposedly the pain of migraine stems from excessively dilated and pulsating cranial arteries of the scalp and dura mater (the tough membrane covering the brain). Ergotamine *constricts* blood vessels, so the theory goes, and thereby prevents pulsating vessels from triggering nearby pain receptors. More particularly, ergotamine produces this constriction by contracting the muscle composing the arterial walls. Likewise, ergonovine contracts the muscle composing the uterus, in this instance the desired effect being to clamp shut this hollow organ and to stop the bleeding. Thus, ergotamine and ergonovine are potent contractors of vascular and visceral muscle and in *toxic* doses produce serious and often irreparable damage.

Ergotism is either acute or chronic, depending on the size of the dose. The acute form relates to a large single dose, and the chronic form to small repeated doses. Bread-borne ergotism is almost always chronic because of the typically minute amounts of ergot present in contaminated flour. In this country, anyway, acute ergotism almost always results from an overdose of an ergot drug (ergotamine, ergonovine, and so on). The acute picture consists of nausea, vomiting, diarrhea, dizziness, tightness in the chest, labored breathing, visual disturbances, prickling sensations, numbness, and, in severe cases, loss of consciousness. Chronic poisoning, however, takes one of two general forms, the convulsive and the gangrenous. Rarely do both occur in the same person, and, as a rule, one form predominates during an epidemic. In the convulsive type, the symptoms are depression, weakness, drowsiness, headache, dizziness, itching, painful cramps in the extremities, and, in severe cases, epileptiform convulsions and paralysis. The gangrenous type is marked by headache, nausea, vomiting, diarrhea, chest pain, irregular heart, and swelling and inflammation of one or more extremities. After the swelling, there may be blisters, redness, cyanosis (blueness of the skin) and finally gangrene. Sometimes there is no preliminary swelling and the gangrene is said to be of the "dry" kind. The hand, the fingers, the feet, the toes, the ears, or nose can be involved and destroyed. What happens, here, of course, is easy enough to explain; that is, the vessels are so constricted that the tissues in the affected parts die from a lack of

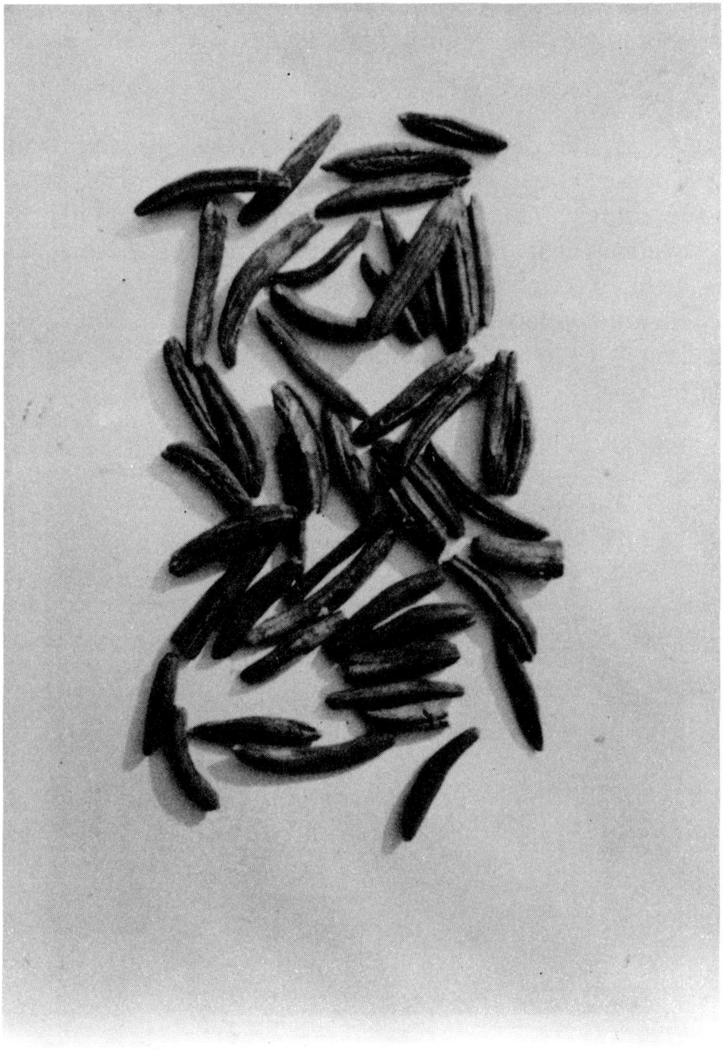

The toxic fungus, ergot (*Claviceps purpurea*).

blood. The serious phase of ergotism may persist for several weeks, with convalescence requiring six months to a year. In fatal cases death usually occurs in a few days after the onset of symptoms.

The treatment in the acute case consists of removing the toxic material by gastric lavage and catharsis and the allaying of the signs and symptoms; the management of the chronic case is almost entirely symptomatic. Amyl nitrite (by inhalation), nitroglycerine (under the tongue), and papaverine (by injection) are useful in combating arterial spasms, and short-acting barbiturates are useful in controlling convulsions. . . . The "best medicine," needless to say, is the proper processing of grain at the mill.

15
Parsnips

For corrupting Athenian youth, the great Socrates was put to death by poison hemlock. Or then again, was it *water* hemlock? Both plants are extremely dangerous and probably kill at least two or three of their dozen or so victims a year.

Poison hemlock (botanically, *Conium maculatum*) is a rather conspicuous biennial weed found in gardens and fields along the roadside. It reaches up to five feet or more in height and its hollow, purplish-spotted stem gives rise to parsleylike leaves (hence, the name "poison parsley") and small, white and grayish green flowers borne on umbrellalike stalks. The roots resemble those of parsnip and when cut exude a juice with the odor of parsnip and related edible plants. The fresh leaves, too, yield such a juice, all of which nicely explains why the philosopher's poison has been mistakenly eaten for parsnip, horseradish, artichoke, sweet cicely, and wild carrot, to name a few possibilities. Understandably, most poisonings occur in children (and cattle). The plant's active principle is coniine, a highly toxic, oily chemical present in the leaves, fruit, and older roots. Coniine is also present throughout the tissues of fools' parsley (*Aethusa cynapium*) and poisonings occur among those who are indeed fooled.

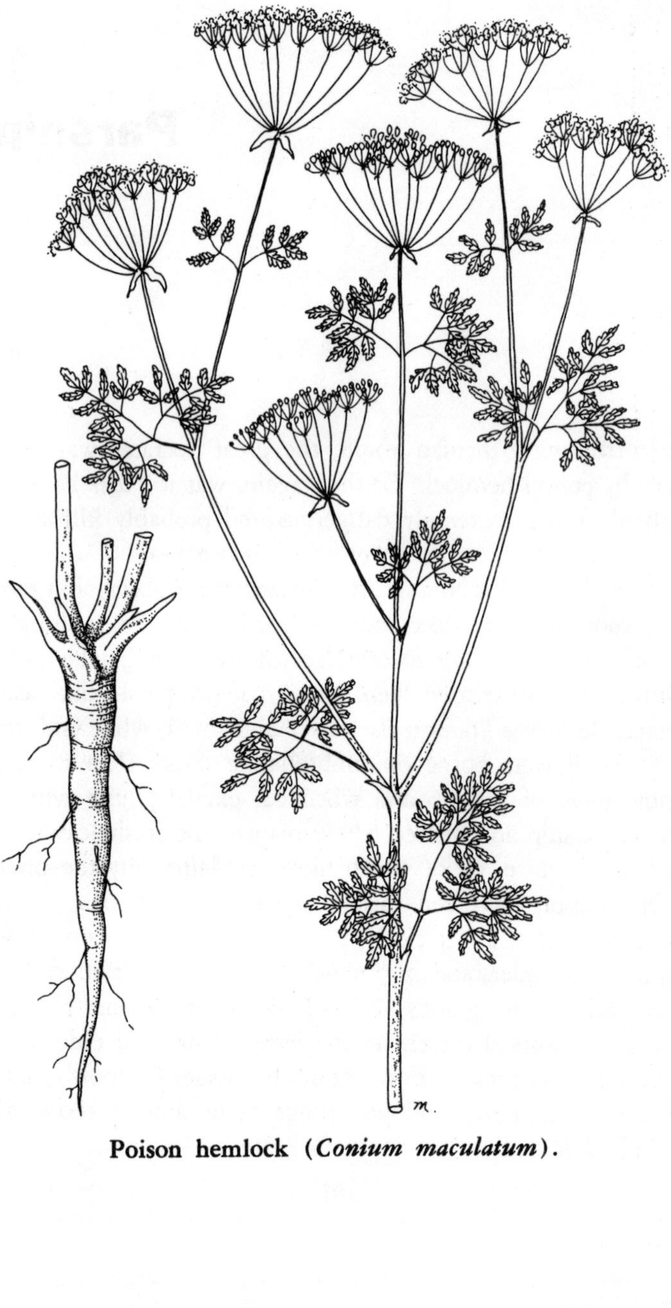

Poison hemlock (*Conium maculatum*).

Coniine attacks the body in much the same manner as the South American poison curare, the major site of action being at the nerve endings. In brief, the poison prevents the nerve impulse from bridging the gap between said endings and muscle and thereby brings about a generalized paralysis. (An interesting mark of distinction between coniine and curare relates to the influence of gastrointestinal juice; the juice readily deactivates curare, but not coniine.) The usual picture of poisoning following the eating of poison hemlock or fools' parsley includes weakness, languor, drunken gait, dilated pupils, drooping eyelids, double vision, difficulty in swallowing, tremors, coldness of the extremities, muscular weakness, and, terminally, respiratory paralysis. The intellect remains clear up until the end; somewhat surprisingly, nausea and vomiting may or may not occur.

With early and adequate treatment the victim has a very good chance to pull through, probably better than ten to one. Vomiting and gastric lavage do much to evacuate the still unabsorbed poison and together amount to the most specific emergency tactic. Once coniine is absorbed, however, all therapeutic measures become purely symptomatic because nothing can be done to deactivate the poison in the blood and tissues. Keeping the patient warm is important and the giving of caffeine, benzedrine, and other stimulants affords some relief. Tea and coffee are useful if they can be swallowed. Oxygen and artificial respiration are lifesaving in severe cases.

Water hemlock, a perennial weed of moist and swampy places, is also known as cowbane, beaver poison, and musquash root; the botanist calls it *Cicuta maculata.* The stem is shiny and hollow and, like poison hemlock, often has purple spots. The leaves are coarsely divided into leaflets, the flowers are white and small, and the tiny fruits are borne on umbrella-like stalks. The roots resemble parsnip and commonly possess many tuberous rootlets not unlike sweet potatoes; the insidious

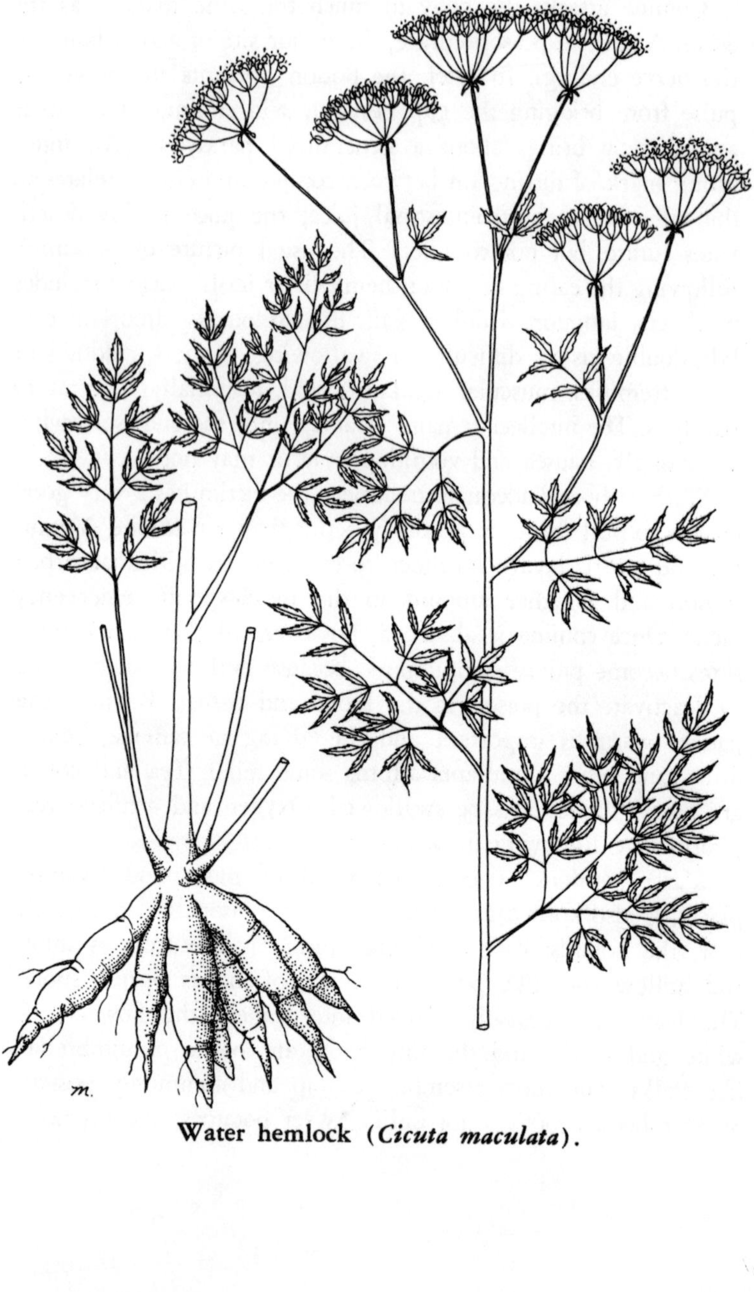

Water hemlock (*Cicuta maculata*).

similarities account for accidental poisoning in adults as well as children. When cut open these roots exude a yellowish aromatic oil containing the poison cicutoxin, one of the most violent substances known to toxicology. To a lesser degree cicutoxin is present in the leaves.

The signs and symptoms commence very soon after eating the plant and run the gamut of what the word "poison" brings to mind. There is burning in the mouth and throat, violent nausea and vomiting, severe abdominal pain, diarrhea, pallor, weakness, labored breathing, mental confusion, writhing movements, and finally convulsions. Especially severe poisonings often lead to the bizarre and ominous opisthotonus, a form of tetanic spasm in which the head and the heels are bent backward and the body forward. Death is from exhaustion and respiratory failure. According to one authoritative source a mouthful of the root can kill a man in 15 minutes, and all references agree on the poor prognosis in severe cases not attended to at the outset—not attended to before a big dose of cicutoxin has passed into the circulation. The first order of business, then, is to evacuate the stomach and prevent this. Less specific measures call for the judicious use of intravenous sedatives, such as Pentothal, to control convulsions and artificial respiration with oxygen to prevent suffocation.

. . . . All that glitters is not gold and all that smells like parsnip is not parsnip. It could be *Conium maculatum* or, worse yet, *Cicuta maculata.*

16
Rhubarb

Oxalic acid is a crystalline compound known to the laboratory and household since time immemorial. It has been used as a disinfectant, cleansing agent for automobile radiators and metals in general, as a laundry bleach, and in textile finishing and cleaning. Both the acid and its salts (namely, potassium oxalate) are poisonous, and a fraction of an ounce can kill. They poison and kill in a most precise and interesting way, basically by reacting with the calcium dissolved in the blood to form *insoluble* calcium oxalate. Only *soluble* calcium can enter the cells, which means in effect that although calcium is still present it is not available to the tissues. Nervous and muscle tissues are especially embarrassed by this event and immediately go awry. Additionally, calcium oxalate may clog and plug the microscopic tubules composing the kidney, and, in the case of the acid, there may be extensive corrosive action. After all, oxalic acid does dissolve rust.

Children and adults may accidentally ingest toxic quantities of oxalic acid. Children and adults have also been poisoned by the oxalates housed in the *leaves* of the common garden rhubarb (pie plant), the child at play and the adult in the quest

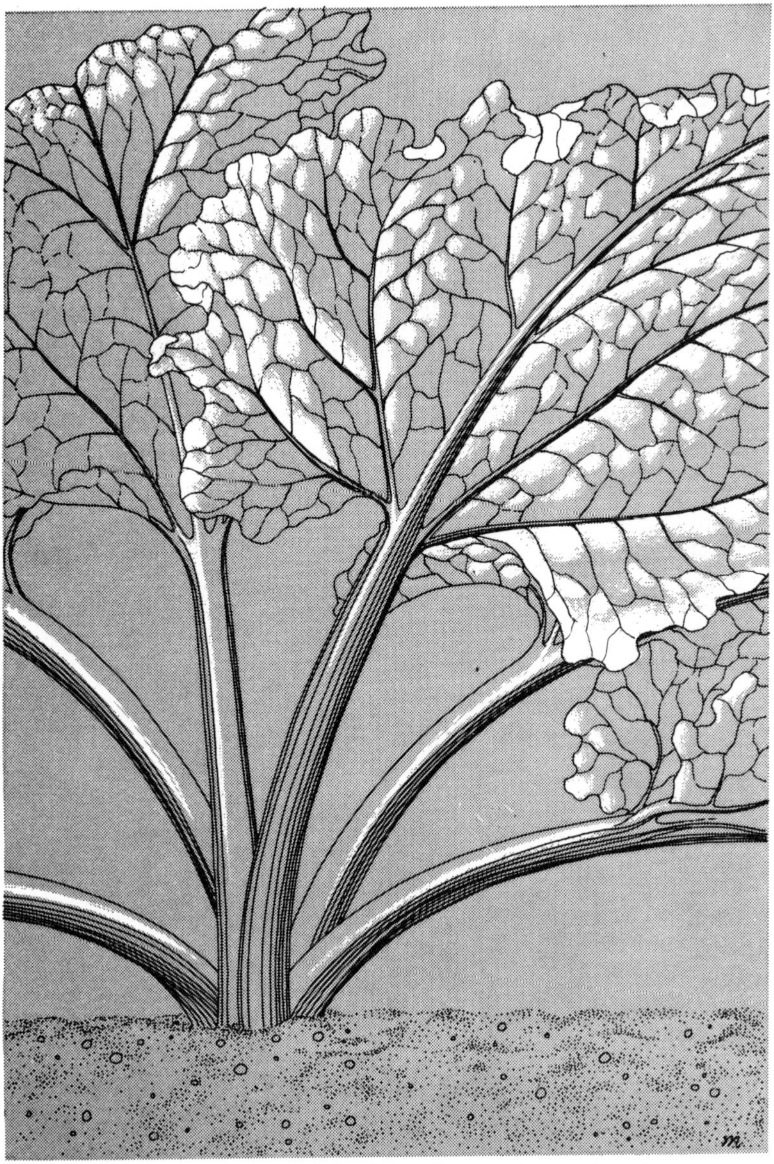

Common garden rhubarb (*Rheum rhaponticum*).

of "greens." The cooked and sweetened stalks of this plant do indeed make a most delicious pie, but the leaves cause vomiting, severe abdominal pain, weakness, and muscle cramps. The eating of large amounts may cause convulsions, coma, and sometimes death. The eating of a single leaf has been known to kill the small child. Death may occur within minutes, or days later—after apparent recovery!—from kidney failure. On-the-spot treatment centers on induced vomiting and the use of antidotes to produce *insoluble* oxalates, in which form they cannot be absorbed into the blood. Milk of magnesia and Epsom salt yield insoluble magnesium oxalate, and milk, lime water, or even ordinary chalk, yield the insoluble calcium oxalate. Management at the hospital includes gastric lavage and the intravenous administration of calcium gluconate to provide the tissues with soluble calcium. The latter measure, especially, can very well mean the difference between life and death. . . . Best of all, enjoy the stalks, but leave the leaves alone!

17
Tea

Jimsonweed (aliases Jamestown weed, thorn apple, stramonium) is a coarse, annual herb having large trumpet-shaped white or purplish flowers and prickly fruit. The latter turns brown when ripe and spills out several small darkish, kidney-shaped seeds. These and the leaves and roots are highly poisonous because of their content of potent alkaloids (hyoscyamine, scopolamine, and atropine, among others). Actually, atropine and scopolamine are valuable drugs but they must be used under close medical supervision and in extremely *small* doses.

Poisonings have occurred after ingestion of the seeds, of tea made from the leaves, and of tomatoes grafted to a host jimsonweed. The tea is a folk-remedy "pick me up" and cure-all, especially for asthma. True enough, atropine relieves asthma, and some doctors do prescribe it for this purpose, but such a tea not uncommonly amounts to too much of a good thing. Alas, poisoning can be experienced merely by handling the leaves!

The symptoms are spectacular. The first are burning and dryness of the mouth, intense thirst, and visual disturbances; the pupils are widely dilated and do not react to light and darkness. Weakness, giddiness, a staggering gait, mental confusion,

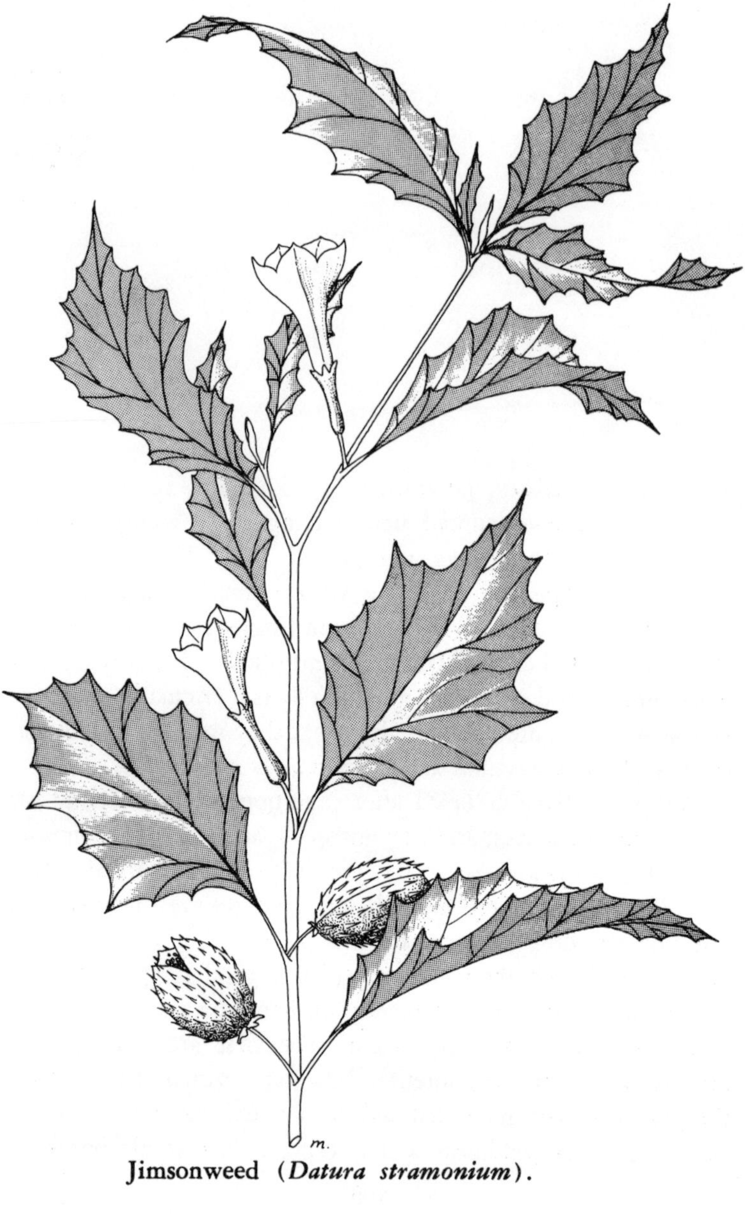

Jimsonweed (*Datura stramonium*).

excitement and delirium then ensue, and in fatal cases convulsions and coma precede death. Evacuation of the poison via gastric lavage and catharsis may be the only therapy necessary in the early stage. A quiet, dark room is essential and sedatives should be given to control excitement and convulsions. In later stages of the poisoning, however, when excitement gives way to depression, large or even moderate doses of sedatives can be dangerous. Here stimulants and artificial respiration (with oxygen) are called for. Sometimes all measures fail . . . a high price for a cup of tea.

18 Peaches

Hydrocyanic acid (prussic acid) is one of the most deadly and probably the most *rapidly* acting poisons known.* Ten grains of the stuff can kill in a minute's time! And the way it exercises its lethalness is the quintessence of all that toxicology has to offer—the destruction of the cell's oxidative enzymes. That is, cyanide poisoning is fundamentally a case of cellular asphyxia.

Almost no one encounters hydrocyanic acid in daily affairs, so what a surprise it is to discover that this lethal chemical occurs in bitter almonds and the seeds and pits of many fruits, notably peaches, plums, and cherries. For the sake of accuracy, though, hydrocyanic acid does not occur per se, but rather as a non-poisoning substance called amygdalin. In the presence of warm water a chemical reaction ensues, and amygdalin breaks down into an assortment of things, *including* the acid. An ounce of cherry pits yields enough to poison an adult or kill a small child. Six ounces of the pits could kill anyone!

Small doses produce vomiting, diarrhea, mental confusion, dizziness, headache, labored breathing, weakness, glassy protrud-

* Hydrocyanic acid is an aqueous solution of hydrogen cyanide, the gas used in the *gas chamber*.

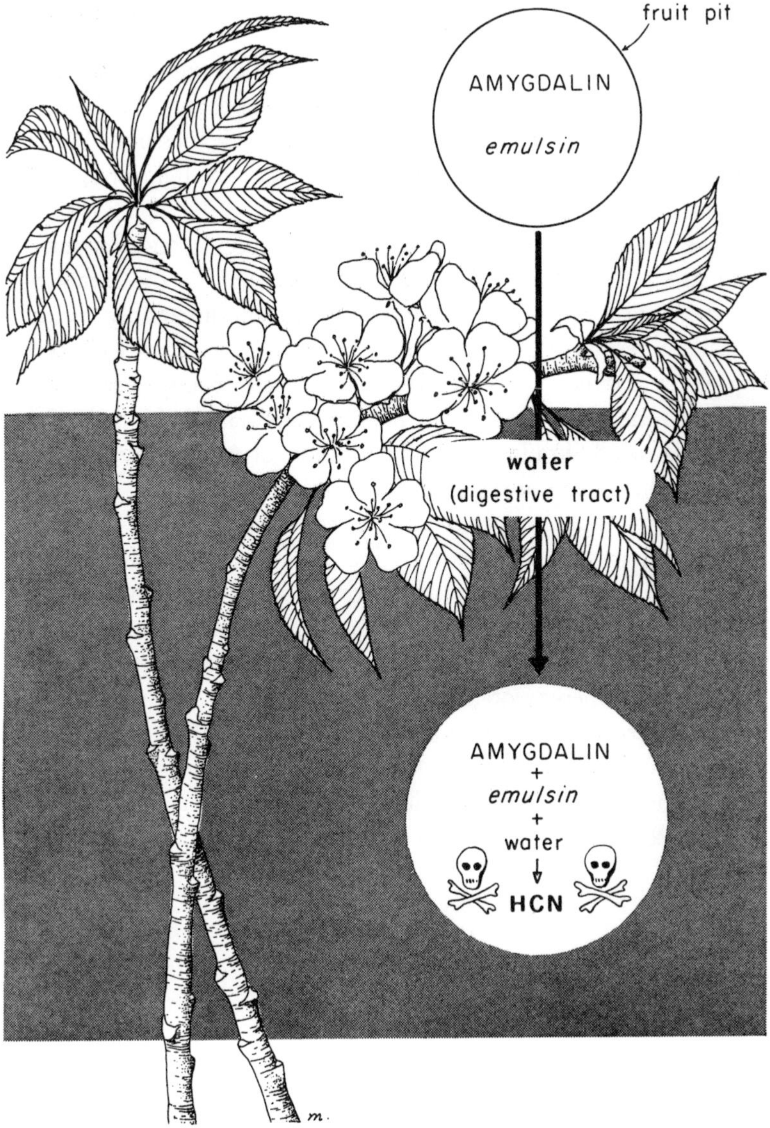

Bitter almonds and the pits of many fruits (notably peaches, plums, and cherries) contain amygdalin and the enzyme emulsin. In the presence of *water* emulsin converts amygdalin into the deadly hydrocyanic acid (HCN).

ing eyes, dilated pupils, pale face, frothing at the mouth, unconsciousness, violent convulsions, stupor, and coma. The breath has the haunting odor of bitter almond or peach blossoms. With large doses there is sudden death, as if struck by lightning, and the victim may never utter a cry.

The treatment of cyanide poisoning is specific and dramatic and often lifesaving if instituted immediately. In the instance of swallowed pits or seeds prompt treatment invariably yields excellent results. Vomiting should be induced at once, followed by gastric lavage at the hospital. Then pearls of amyl nitrite are broken, one at a time, in a handkerchief and held over the patient's nose. Simultaneously, a solution of sodium nitrite and sodium thiosulfate are shot into a vein, and this to be repeated if poisoning signs reappear or recovery is slow. What happens here is chemically fascinating. The nitrites convert the hemoglobin of the red cells to a derivative (called methemoglobin) with such an affinity for cyanide that it prevents the latter from entering the cells. The tactic now is to gradually convert the worthless methemoglobin back into hemoglobin and a *nontoxic* cyanide derivative which is eventually excreted. This is the purpose and function of the sodium thiosulfate. Few poisonings can be handled in a more tailor-made fashion. . . . But this is no excuse for thinking lightly of pits and seeds and stones.

19
Lemonade

Food contaminated with noxious chemicals in sufficient amounts to cause *acute* poisoning is not a common occurrence, but it does indeed occur. Further, there is the classic instance where a poison is mistaken for food or where a poison has been purposely added to food—a well-established practice among the criminal element of yesteryears. For the most part, the situation today boils down to sodium fluoride, metals, and insecticides.

Sodium fluoride, one of the most poisonous substances known, presents a special problem because (A) it resembles baking soda, baking powder, and the like and (B) it is often used to exterminate cockroaches. More to the point, the chemical turns up frequently in the kitchen and the cook makes a mistake. And the consequences can be horrendous, as they were the day a kitchen helper at Oregon State Hospital mistook the "roach powder" for powdered milk and added about 17 pounds of it to a 10 gallon mixture of scrambled eggs. The upshot was 263 poisonings and 47 deaths! From this episode and similar tragedies the lethal dose is known to be about three grams, or one-tenth ounce.

As to the mechanism of fluoride poisoning, there appears to

be an interplay between a calcium upset and enzyme interference. In the test tube, sodium fluoride reacts with *soluble* calcium compounds to produce *insoluble* calcium fluoride; if this occurs in blood, and there is much evidence that it does, calcium is thereby cut off from the cells. (Only *soluble* substances can pass through the cell membrane.) Also, the test tube demonstrates that the chemical interferes with a number of enzymes (chemical "spark plugs") responsible for the production of cellular energy. In sum, sodium fluoride amounts to a "protoplasmic poison," and this is just what many toxicologists call it.

The onset of fluoride poisoning is a matter of minutes after ingestion, and in the instance of lethal amounts death occurs within eight hours unless promptly treated. The symptoms consist of salivation, bloody vomiting, abdominal cramps, weakness, heart failure, shallow breathing and eventually respiratory failure. Epileptiform convulsions may occur and blood may be present in the urine as a result of severe damage to the kidneys. Induced vomiting and the giving of "calcium" (as calcium chloride, calcium gluconate, lime water, or copious milk) will do much to convert the poison to the relatively innocuous *calcium* fluoride. This first-aid measure can be lifesaving. At the hospital, gastric lavage is carried out with calcium chloride and the patient given calcium gluconate intravenously. Artificial respiration, sedatives, and other supportive treatment are given as needed.

Metal poisoning invariably involves the preparation or storage of food, especially *acidic* beverages, in receptacles composed of or lined with toxic metals. Lead, zinc, copper, and cadmium are the usual culprits. What happens is that enough of the metal is leeched out of the receptacle or container to produce an acute gastroenteritis. To cite actual cases: Lead poisoning has resulted from serving "soda pop" in lead-glazed pottery; copper poisoning has resulted from keeping root beer in copper utensils; and zinc poisoning has resulted from making lemonade in zinc (galvanized) coolers. Of most toxicological concern, however, is *cadmium* poisoning.

Cadmium is a soft, bluish-white metal used in fatigue-resistant alloys, solders, nickel-cadmium storage batteries, and in the plating of metals, which accounts for its involvement in food poisoning. At one time cadmium-plated utensils, metal pitchers, ice-cube trays, and the like, were very much in vogue; when acid foods or liquids are stored or prepared in these enough of the metal is dissolved away to produce severe poisoning and even death. As little as 10 milligrams, not much more than a large speck, can cause marked symptoms. Made to order for this type of poisoning are fruit juices and lemonade, and these beverages are indeed the usual offenders. Although the law prohibits the use and manufacture of cadmium cooking utensils, refrigerator pitchers, trays, and so on, they are still in evidence and still responsible for sporadic outbreaks of poisoning both here and abroad.

The onset of cadmium poisoning is usually a matter of minutes and the symptoms usually last for 24 hours. These consist of violent gastric and abdominal cramps, salivation, vomiting, diarrhea, nausea, headache, muscular pain, shivering, dizziness, sensory disturbances in the hands and arms and sometimes convulsions. In the fatal case death is due to respiratory depression. Treatment centers on gastric lavage with milk or egg white, catharsis, artificial respiration, and the intravenous administration of a "systemic antidote" by the name of calcium disodium edetate. This agent does a good job detoxifying absorbed cadmium, but it is not kind to the kidneys, meaning that it must be used judiciously with this in mind.

Another utensil of toxicological interest and concern is old gray-enameled ware; often contained in the binding between the enamel and metal is antimony—an element about as toxic

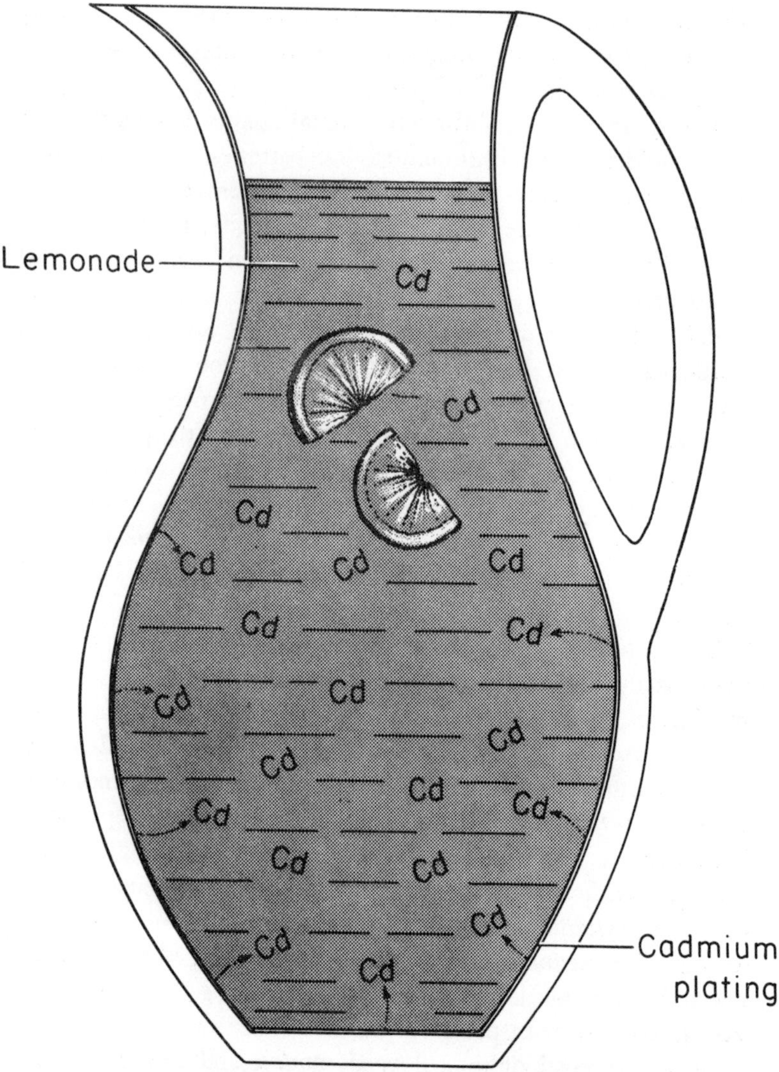

The acid in fruit drinks dissolves away cadmium in cadmium-plated utensils—*time* permitting, a sufficient amount to cause poisoning.

as arsenic. Antimony poisoning, though rare, has resulted from cooking in such utensils, and, as in the case of cadmium, acidic liquids pose a special danger; that is, there may be just enough citric acid in the lemonade to dissolve away a toxic dose of antimony. Generally, the symptoms appear within a few minutes to one hour, and the first to appear are constriction of the throat and intense gastric pain. Next follows projectile vomiting of "rice-water" fluid, which becomes sticky and bloody, and profuse diarrhea with bloody stools. Coma and convulsions may occur and total collapse may ensue. Treatment entails gastric lavage, artificial respiration, morphine to control pain, fluids to counteract dehydration, and injections of dimercaprol to detoxify the antimony that has been absorbed into the blood. Prompt treatment bodes a favorable prognosis.

Among other offbeat involvements are "well-water poisoning" and the "Chinese-restaurant syndrome." In some localities well water contains high enough concentrations of nitrates to cause poisoning, particularly when the water is used in making the baby's formula. In one classic outbreak in Minnesota, there were 139 cases (among infants) with 14 deaths. Poisoning is rare after six months of age. Presumably, the nitrates are converted to nitrites by bacterial action in the intestines, and nitrites are known to change hemoglobin (in the red cells) to methemoglobin, a form of hemoglobin that does not combine with and carry oxygen. The upshot is "cellular asphyxia." The patient will have cyanosis (blueness of the skin), which begins around the lips, spreads to the fingers and toes, the face, and eventually to the entire body. Additional features are gastrointestinal upset, respiratory and circulatory failure, and in severe poisoning coma and death may result. The treatment of choice is methylene blue given intravenously, an antidote that converts the worthless methemoglobin back to normal, oxygen-carrying hemoglobin. Other important measures include the use of stimulants, oxygen, and blood transfusions.

The so-called "Chinese-restaurant syndrome," now a recognized poisoning, occurs when susceptible persons ingest large amounts (5 grams or more) of monosodium glutamate, a major condiment in Chinese food. The symptoms generally begin 10 to 20 minutes after the meal and include palpitations, headache, dizziness, flushing, severe pain about the eyes and temporal areas of the head, and tingling sensations in the back of the neck, upper back, arms, and chest. These manifestations fluctuate in intensity and usually disappear in an hour or so. Although no fatalities or lasting effects have been reported, the experience is frightening and obviously to be guarded against once the susceptibility has been identified.

Bibliography

Books

Anderson, W. A. D., and Scotti, T. M., *Synopsis of Pathology,* 7th ed. St. Louis: The C. V. Mosby Co., 1968.

Bailey, W. R., and Scott, E., *Diagnostic Microbiology: A Laboratory Manual.* St. Louis: The C. V. Mosby Co., 1970.

Boyd, W., *An Introduction to the Study of Disease,* 6th ed. Philadelphia: Lea and Febiger, 1971.

Boyd, W., *Textbook of Pathology,* 8th ed. Philadelphia: Lea and Febiger, 1970.

Brooks, S. M., *Integrated Basic Science,* 3rd ed. St. Louis: The C. V. Mosby Co., 1970.

———. *A Programmed Introduction to Microbiology,* 2nd ed. St. Louis: The C. V. Mosby Co., 1973.

Burrows, W., *Textbook of Microbiology,* 19th ed. Philadelphia: The W. B. Saunders Co., 1968.

Carpenter, P. L., *Microbiology,* 2nd ed. Philadelphia: The W. B. Saunders Co., 1967.

Cecil-Loeb Textbook of Medicine, 13th ed. Philadelphia: The W. B. Saunders Co., 1971.

Dack, G., *Food Poisoning,* 3rd ed. Chicago: University of Chicago Press, 1956.

Elveback, L. R., *Epidemiology.* New York: Macmillan, 1970.

Frazier, W. C., *Food Microbiology,* 2nd ed. New York: McGraw Hill Book Co., 1967.

Gebhardt, L. P., *Microbiology,* 4th ed. St. Louis: The C. V. Mosby Co., 1970.

Goldbirth, S. A. (editor), *Exploration in Future Food Processing Techniques.* Cambridge: Massachusetts Institute of Technology Press, 1963.

Goodman, L. S., and Gilman, A., *The Pharmacological Basis of Therapeutics,* 3rd ed. New York: The Macmillan Co., 1965.

Harvey, A. M., Johns, R. J., Owens, A. H., and Ross, R. S., *The Principles and Practice of Medicine,* 17th ed. New York: Appleton-Century-Crofts, 1968.

Holvey, D. N. (editor), *The Merck Manual,* 12th ed. Rahway: Merck, Sharp and Dohme Research Laboratories, 1972.

Lucas, G. H. W., *The Symptoms and Treatment of Acute Poisoning.* New York: The Macmillan Co., 1953.

Muenscher, W. C., *Poisonous Plants in the United States.* New York: The Macmillan Co., 1939.

Robbins, S. L., *Textbook of Pathology,* 3rd ed. Philadelphia: W. B. Saunders Co., 1967.

Slanetz, L. W., Chichester, C. O., Ganfin, A. R., and Ordal, Z. J. (editors), *Microbiological Quality of Food.* New York: Academic Press, Inc., 1963.

Smith, A. L., *Microbiology and Pathology,* 9th ed. St. Louis: The C. V. Mosby Co., 1968.

Smith, D. T., et al, *Zinsser Microbiology,* 14th ed. New York: Appleton-Century-Crofts, 1968.

Sollmann, T., *A Manual of Pharmacology,* 8th ed. Philadelphia: The W. B. Saunders Co., 1957.

Stanier, R. Y., Doudoroff, M., and Adelberg, E. A., *The Microbial World,* 2nd ed. Englewood Cliffs: Prentice-Hall, Inc., 1963.

Thienes, C. H., and Haley, T. J., *Clinical Toxicology,* 5th ed. Philadelphia: Lea and Febiger, 1970.

Top, F. H., *Communicable and Infectious Diseases,* 6th ed. St. Louis: The C. V. Mosby Co., 1968.

von Oettingen, W. F., *Poisoning,* 2nd ed. Philadelphia: The W. B. Saunders Co., 1962.

Wheeler, M. F., and Volk, W. A., *Basic Microbiology,* 2nd ed. Philadelphia: J. B. Lippincott Co., 1969.

Journals

Adelson, L., "Common Poisons." *American Journal of Clinical Pathology, 22:*509, 1952.

Arena, J. M., "Diagnosis and Treatment of Poisoning." *Clinical Symposia, 12:*1, 1960.

Baader, et al, "Cadmium Poisoning." *Industrial Medicine and Surgery, 21:*427, 1952.

Barrett-Conner, E., "Shigellosis in the Adult." *Journal of the American Medical Association, 198:*717, 1966.

Benson, H. W., "Rhubarb Poisoning." *Journal of the American Medical Association, 73:*1152, 1919.

Benson, J., "Poisonous Fish." *Forensic Science, 1:*119, 1956.

Bentler, E., "L-Dopa and Favism." *Blood, 36:*523, 1970.

Burr, H. K., and Elliott, R. P., "Quality and Safety in Frozen Foods." *Journal of the American Medical Association, 174:*1178, 1962.

Bicknell, W. J., and Collins, J. C., "The Paralytic Shellfish Poisoning Incident in Massachusetts." (A paper read before the American Public Health Association on November 13, 1972.)

Center for Disease Control, "Foodborne Outbreaks." *Annual Summary,* 1969.

———, "Foodborne Outbreaks." *Annual Summary,* 1970.

———, "Foodborne Outbreaks," *Annual Summary,* 1971.

———, "Reported Incidence of Notifiable Diseases in the United States, 1971." *Morbidity and Mortality, 20:*53, 1972.

Cheever, F. S., "The Acute Diarrheal Disease of Bacterial Origin." *Bulletin of New York Academy of Medicine, 31:*611–26, 1955.

Clay, A. L., "Milk Sickness." *Illinois Medical Journal, 26:*103, 1914.

Cotter, L. H., and Cotter, B. H., "Cadmium Poisoning." *Archives of Industrial Hygiene, 3:*495, 1951.

Couch, J. F. J., "Milk Poisoning." *Agricultural Research, 40:*649, 1930.

Dack, G. M., "Current Status of Therapy in Microbial Food Poisoning." *Journal of the American Medical Association, 172:*929, 1960.

Dack, G. M., et al, "Feeding Tests on Human Volunteers with Enterococci and Tyramine." *Journal of Infectious Diseases, 85:*131, 1949.

Editorial, "Milk Sickness." *Journal of the American Medical Association, 87:*555, 1925.

Editorial, "Modern Conditions Seem to Suit Salmonellae." *Journal of the American Medical Association, 222:*9, 1972.

Editorial, "Poisonous Fish." *Journal of the American Medical Association, 163:*118, 1957.

Friberg, L., "Cadmium Poisoning." *Archives of Industrial Hygiene, 1:*458, 1950.

Galbraith, N., "Staphylococcal Food Poisoning." *Practitioner, 195:* 18–26, 1965.

Halstead, B. W., "Fish Poisonings—Their Diagnosis, Pharmacology and Treatment." *Clinical Pharmacology and Therapeutics, 5:*615, 1964.

Harrison, D. C., et al, "Mushroom Poisoning in Five Patients." *American Journal of Medicine, 38:*787, 1963.

Hutton, J. E., "Fava Bean Poisoning." *Journal of the American Medical Association, 109:*1618, 1937.

Johnston, R. W., Feldman, J., and Sullivan, R., "Botulism from Canned Tuna Fish." *Public Health Reports, 78:*7, 1963.

Kautter, D. A., "Botulism." *Morbidity and Mortality, 13:*1, 1964.

———, "Clostridium Botulinum Type E in Smoked Fish." *Journal of Food Science, 29:*6, 1964.

———, "Type E Botulism." *Journal of the American Medical Association,* Feb. 15, 1964.

Kilborn, L. G., et al, "Fluoride Poisoning." *Canadian Medical Association Journal, 62:*135, 1950.

Koenig, M. G., et al, "Clinical and Laboratory Observations in Type E Botulism in Man." *Medicine, 43:*517, 1964.

———, "Type B Botulism in Man." *American Journal of Medicine, 42:*208, 1967.

Meyers, K. F., "Food Poisoning." *New England Journal of Medicine, 249:*765, 1953.

Meyers, K. F., et al, "Shellfish Poisoning." *Preventive Medicine, 2:* 365, 1928.

Miller, W. A., "The Microbiology of Self-Service, Pre-Packaged Fresh Pork Sausage." *Journal of Milk Food Technology, 27:*1, 1964.

Mitchell, J. E., and Mitchell, F. N., "Jimsonweed Poisoning." *Journal of Pediatrics, 47:*227, 1955.

National Center for Health Statistics, "Acute Conditions." *Vital and Health Statistics,* Series 10–No. 77, August, 1972.

Pare, C. M. B., and Sandler, M., "Zinc Poisoning." *Royal Army Medical Corps, 100:*320, 1954.

Rabinowitch, I. M., "Fluoride Poisoning." *Canadian Medical Association Journal, 52:*345, 1945.

Rogers, D. E., "Botulism: Vintage 1963." Editorial. *Annals of Internal Medicine, 61:*581, 1964.

Rosen, A. P., and Scanlan, J. J., "Favism." *New England Journal of Medicine, 239:*367, 1948.

Russo, G., et al, "Hemolytic Crises of Favism in Sicilian Females Heterozygous for G-6PD Deficiency." *Pediatrics,* Vol. 49, 1972.

Smith, J. P., "Cadmium Poisoning." *Journal of Pathology and Bacteriology, 80:*287, 1960.

Splittstoesser, D. F., and Wettergreen, W. A., "The Significance of Coliforms in Frozen Vegetables." *Journal of Milk Food Technology, 27:*134, 1964.

Taylor, J., "Salmonella Food Poisoning." *Practitioner, 195:*12–17, 1965.

Walsh, E. W., "Milk Poisoning." *Journal of the American Medical Association, 87:*555, 1925.

Index